MW01227082

Rational
EMOTIVE
BEHAVIOUR
THERAPY
Integrated

Rational
EMOTIVE
BEHAVIOUR
THERAPY
Integrated

Anjali Joshi
K.M. Phadke

Los Angeles | London | New Delhi
Singapore | Washington DC | Melbourne

First published in 2018 by

 SAGE Publications India Pvt Ltd
B1/I-1 Mohan Cooperative Industrial Area
Mathura Road, New Delhi 110 044, India
www.sagepub.in

SAGE Publications Inc
2455 Teller Road
Thousand Oaks, California 91320, USA

SAGE Publications Ltd
1 Oliver's Yard, 55 City Road
London EC1Y 1SP, United Kingdom

SAGE Publications Asia-Pacific Pte Ltd
3 Church Street
#10-04 Samsung Hub
Singapore 049483

Published by Vivek Mehra for SAGE Publications India Pvt Ltd, typeset in 10/12 pt Times New Roman by Fidus Design Pvt. Ltd., Chandigarh and printed at Chaman Enterprises, New Delhi.

Library of Congress Cataloging-in-Publication Data

Names: Joshi, Anjali (Psychologist) author. | Phadke, K.M., author.
Title: Rational emotive behaviour therapy integrated / Anjali Joshi, K.M. Phadke.
Description: New Delhi; Thousand Oaks, California: SAGE Publications, 2018. |
    Includes bibliographical references and index.
Identifiers: LCCN 2017043739| ISBN 9789352805129 (hb) | ISBN 9789352805143 (e-pub 2.0) |
    ISBN 9789352805136 (ebook)
Subjects: MESH: Psychotherapy, Rational-Emotive
Classification: LCC RC454 | NLM WM 420.5.P8 | DDC 616.89/14—dc23
LC record available at https://lccn.loc.gov/2017043739

ISBN: 978-93-528-0512-9 (HB)

SAGE Team: Abhijit Baroi, Vandana Gupta, Kumar Indra Mishra and Ritu Chopra

To

Rita Khear, our long-time associate
For her unconditional warmth and support!

Thank you for choosing a SAGE product!
If you have any comment, observation or feedback,
I would like to personally hear from you.

Please write to me at **contactceo@sagepub.in**

Vivek Mehra, Managing Director and CEO, SAGE India.

Contents

List of Illustrations

Tables

Figures

Boxes

Preface

Dr Albert Ellis (1913–2007), the eminent American psychologist, is considered to be one of the most influential figures in the field of psychology. He is the originator of Rational Emotive Behaviour Therapy (REBT), a leading cognitive behavioural approach to counselling and psychotherapy. By inventing REBT, he had not only revolutionized the field of psychotherapy but also instigated the 'cognitive revolution' in psychology.

REBT focuses on reducing emotional and behavioural disturbances and enabling people to lead happier and more fulfilling lives. Since its inception in 1955, REBT has spread very rapidly and has been practised by many professionals such as psychologists, counsellors, psychiatrists, social workers and mental health workers, owing to a significant portion of population suffering from a wide range of psychological disturbances. REBT has been applied to several areas such as education, industry, geriatrics, alcoholism prevention, religion and many more.

Dr Ellis had contributed greatly to REBT's development. He had written and edited more than 75 books, published more than 800 scientific papers and articles, and created over 200 audio cassettes. He continued to write articles and publish books until his death at the age of 93.

This invaluable work by Dr Ellis on REBT inspired us to undertake the challenging task of introducing the theory and practice of REBT to all those who are interested in learning about it. K.M. Phadke, a senior author, is a pioneer of REBT in India. He is a Fellow and Supervisor of the Albert Ellis Institute, New York. He held correspondence with Dr Ellis from 1968 to 2003, and Dr Ellis tirelessly replied to his series of questions. This unusual correspondence is of four bound volumes and consists of 1,351 pages. It has been preserved in the Columbia University Archives after Dr Ellis' death. Phadke's contributions to REBT were acknowledged by Dr Ellis himself and even applauded by him in his autobiography *All Out!*

I, the presenting author of this book, did my doctorate work in the field of REBT and Phadke (the senior author) has been mentoring me for the past 17 years. The study of REBT is the common bond between us that led to the emergence of this book.

This book has a fairly long history, and the journey of this book had many twists and turns. Its origin can be traced to the article 'Dr Albert Ellis: A Rebellious Psychologist', which Phadke wrote in Marathi. It was published in a well-known Marathi weekly in 1981. After almost 17 years, or to be more precise, on 15 May 1998, he wrote a letter to Dr Ellis and informed him that he would write a full-length Marathi book bearing the above title. He then worked on that project for four years but discontinued it due to some difficulties in translating, to his own satisfaction, technical terms into Marathi. This work was later completed by me, and I subsequently published a Marathi volume on it—*Albert Ellis: Vichardarshan.*

The motivation to write this book has emerged from a strong need we felt while conducting training programmes on REBT—to have a book that provides handy information on all the features of REBT. In many discussions, our colleagues and participants too stressed this need. Most of the available REBT books emphasize on a few fundamental features of REBT and generally do not cover all of them. In view of this situation, we felt the necessity to produce valuable literature on REBT, describing it entirely from its origin to applications. It would be a comprehensive handbook on REBT for those who wish to learn or practise it. During our extensive counselling practice of dealing with a variety of clients, we realized the necessity to include in the book a few representative cases of psychological disturbance that will help the readers to understand various components of REBT effortlessly.

Along the same line of thought, Phadke spearheaded the work and completed the first draft in January 2007. This work came to a standstill when Dr Ellis passed away on 24 July 2007. Moreover, the first draft had many limitations. Some of the limitations were caused by the insufficiency of resources at his disposal. The book was silent on many developments of REBT, and many records and references were incomplete because he had no reliable knowledge about them.

The book got a new lease of life in 2013 when I ventured to rewrite this book on the occasion of Dr Ellis' 100th birth anniversary. This work extended for four more years, and the book shaped into its present form. This book is the outcome of prolonged efforts of both of us. It is based on our work on 500 research papers, essays and 75 books written by Dr Ellis.

While working on the present form of the book, I had to completely rewrite a few chapters. I have tried to incorporate the contents from latest publications and have added several topics on new REBT formulations.

I have also included revised and updated information in all the chapters. In doing all this, I have attempted to produce a book that will present a comprehensive picture of the theory and practice of REBT as well as an overview of Dr Ellis' work on its development.

This is probably the only book on REBT having all-inclusive information about its origin, historical development, philosophical foundation and vivid applications. The book serves three purposes. First, you will get acquainted with Dr Ellis and his main contributions to the field of psychotherapy. Second, it will help you understand the causes of some of the emotional and behavioural problems and some ways to overcome them. Third, it seeks to offer a handy reference to experienced professionals as well as act as a helpful guide to beginners who wish to know REBT in depth.

Since the subject area of the book is REBT, it covers the fields of psychology, counselling, psychotherapy and mental health. It provides multiple insights into your own cognitions, emotions and behaviour. It aims to help you reduce your psychological disturbance and live your life happily. Moreover, the book provides psychologically disturbed individuals with many answers they seek and can help everyone feel better about themselves and deal with their lives more effectively. It will be useful to you if you are keen on self-development, and to professionals belonging to a variety of fields such as mental health, medicine, teaching, social work and parenting.

Let us briefly summarize what has been covered in this book. It is organized into 10 chapters, and each chapter offers an insight on the various distinctive features of REBT. Chapter 1 unfolds how the foundation of REBT was laid in the professional world by Dr Ellis. Chapter 2 focuses on his life story and the significant events that occurred in his life. Chapter 3 is devoted to the historical development of REBT. In the next three chapters (Chapters 4–6), the framework and theoretical nature of REBT are outlined. Here, we present a detailed description of the A, B and C components as well as an extensive illustration of irrational beliefs. In Chapter 7, we stress REBT as a philosophy of life. In Chapter 8, we iterate how the therapeutic process works and the insights obtained from therapy. Further, in Chapter 9, the cognitive, emotive and behavioural techniques of REBT and their practices are discussed. The book concludes in Chapter 10, by discussing the applications of REBT in a variety of fields. Here, the limitations of REBT are brought out as well.

The book contains two appendices. Both appendices are intended to guide you to work on your own emotional disturbance. They have two forms of disputation—one is solved and the other is for practice.

In order to facilitate your learning process, we have chosen and woven throughout the book three live cases of emotional disturbance suitable for cross-cultural population. They represent the three categories of musturbatory beliefs. These cases are drawn from our clinical experience of common emotional problems presented by counselees and can be found in any culture. Hence, you will identify yourself with the characters to a great extent. Multiple components of REBT are explained with reference to these cases. Hence, in every chapter, you will discover new features of emotional disturbance.

We have adopted an easy-to-read style with the intention to make REBT concepts clear and understandable even for people without any previous knowledge of REBT. We have used generic pronouns such as 'you' throughout the book as we prefer to address you directly. Moreover, please note that we have used the masculine form of the singular pronoun ('he', 'him', and 'his') to refer to human beings of either sex.

We hope that this book stimulates your interest in developing your knowledge of and skills in REBT and that you will find it a handy reference in the future. Finally, we wish to add that we have immensely enjoyed the process of writing this book. Moreover, we realized how little we could capture from Dr Ellis' mammoth work on REBT, in spite of having lived in the Ellisian world for ages!

Anjali Joshi

Acknowledgements

We would like to express our deepest gratitude to the late Dr Albert Ellis for making available invaluable material on REBT. The 75 odd books and 500 odd papers that he sent to K.M. Phadke during the 36 years of their correspondence is the primary foundation of this book. This book may not have been written without these resources.

We would also like to thank Rita Khear, whose efforts in typing the manuscript were of great help.

Anay Joshi has also been of inestimable help as he meticulously scrutinized the manuscript from a language point of view.

We greatly appreciate Dr Satishchandra Kumar's contribution in providing excellent support and advice.

Finally, we express our special gratitude to the SAGE team for their valuable suggestions that enriched the content.

Anjali Joshi
K.M. Phadke

1

The Flag of Rebellion Hoisted

In 1956, a huge annual convention was held in Chicago. Many renowned psychologists, belonging to various fields of psychology, attended it. It was organized by the American Psychological Association (APA), a leading scientific and professional organization representing psychology in the United States of America.

American psychologists often consider this convention as a golden opportunity to expand their professional network. They yearn to present their inventions in these conventions as well as to explore content developed by other researchers. This interaction and update is required for the development of their specialized field of knowledge. These annual conventions are a source of inspiration for new ideas to them and an exposure to a variety of points of views.

This convention was no exception. Some topics were discussed at length, while some were discussed peripherally. Some plenary sessions were received well by the audience and some were not. Some sessions sparked lively questions among the participants. This added flavour to the convention.

One psychologist read his paper in the convention on 31 August 1956. The title of this paper was so unique that it raised many eyebrows. The title was 'Rational Therapy'. This title posed many queries in the minds of participants. They began discussing two prominent questions—'What is this unique system of psychotherapy and why it was unheard so far? Who had the cheek to present a paper bearing such a strange title in the convention of professional psychologists?'

The author and presenter of that paper was not a novice psychologist. He had not only earned his PhD in clinical psychology from Columbia University but also had years of experience in the field of psychotherapy. In addition, this 43-year-old psychologist had many research papers and significant books to his credit. It was difficult for the audience to quickly brush aside his unusual ideas and neglect the contribution of this highbrow professional.

The system of rational therapy put forward by this veteran in the Chicago convention definitely contained some concepts and methods which were enough to give a jolt to the concepts prevalent among psychologists of that time. For example, according to him, it is not necessary to find out the original cause of the client's problem by studying his childhood experiences or by delving too deeply into his unconscious mind. Similarly, there is nothing wrong if you sometimes teach a few relevant things to the client straightway or directly guide him. Therefore, it is necessary to throw away the belief that the psychotherapist *should* never teach anything to the client and that he *should* do his work indirectly and without taking any active role in the process of psychotherapy.

On the contrary, the psychotherapist had better teach the client that in order to resolve his problem, it is necessary to detect the irrational ideas and attitudes currently existing in his mind and then attack and destroy them. As a matter of fact, the main cause of man's emotional disturbance is to be found in the illogical and unrealistic ideas and attitudes currently held by him. Hence, if he acquires the discipline of thinking rationally and realistically, he will be able to live a happy and creative life. Needless to say that in this system of psychotherapy, little importance is given to the interpretation of the client's dreams. In short, the main features of this system of psychotherapy existed at least in a germinal form in the very first paper its founder presented in the Chicago convention in 1956.

Admittedly, this sketchy account of rational therapy, called Rational Emotive Behaviour Therapy (REBT) since 1993, is not enough to understand its nature and scope. These characteristics are not mentioned with the objective of describing its main features in detail. That task will be undertaken subsequently. Here, only a few of its characteristics have been broadly stated. The purpose of doing so is to suggest why the emergence of this new psychotherapeutic system might have shocked the psychological establishment.

Indeed, not only were some techniques of this new system of psychotherapy unique but also bound to be considered shocking and iconoclastic by psychotherapists in the 1950s. Because, during those days, the diagnostic and therapeutic methods of analysing the childhood experiences of the client, digging up the information buried in his unconscious mind and interpreting his dreams were adopted by practically all the psychotherapists. In other words, the customary methods of psychotherapy were closely akin to the psychoanalytic methods used by Sigmund Freud and his followers. The psychotherapists who were following Carl Rogers believed that directly or indirectly teaching something to the client and openly giving him advice was detrimental to the effectiveness of psychotherapy.

In such a climate, when the founder of REBT gave the first public presentation of his new brand of psychotherapy at the Annual Convention of the APA in Chicago in 1956, he hoisted the flag of rebellion. This new system of psychotherapy, however, had actually begun to take shape in its founder's mind since 1953 and had been used by him to treat his clients since 1955. In 1958, he published a paper titled 'Rational Psychotherapy' in the *Journal of General Psychology*, a very reputed periodical in the field of psychology (Ellis, 1958).

Who is the man that raised the flag of rebellion by founding this new system of psychotherapy? How did he give birth and rear his brainchild? How has he harnessed the ability to write and speak in order to spread his message throughout the world? What price has he paid for his rebelliousness? What is the outcome of his relentless efforts to develop and practice his brand of psychotherapy for more than 45 years? How did this psychotherapy get recognized globally by professionals around the world? What is its contribution? How can this psychotherapy help the common man?

This book is written to answer these questions. It will provide you with the insight of your emotional problems and offer constructive guidance to solve them. These objectives will be achieved only if you actively try to understand how the causes and cure of emotional disturbance explained in this book are applicable to your own problems.

Reference

Ellis, A. (1958). Rational psychotherapy. *The Journal of General Psychology, 59*(1), 35–49.

2

Life and Development

The man who created a stir among psychologists by presenting an introductory paper at the Annual Convention of APA, now called the REBT, was none other than Albert Ellis. Knowing something about his life and development may provide valuable insights into his system of psychotherapy and will also help you to know how he was, in a way, naturally creating and rearing his system of psychotherapy long before it formally came into existence.

Early Years

Albert was born on 27 September 1913 in Pittsburgh, Pennsylvania. His mother's maiden name was Hettie Hanigbaum who was born in Philadelphia, Pennsylvania. Her parents were Jews who had migrated to the United States of America from Germany. Original name of Albert's father was Henry Oscar Groots. He was born near Vineland, New Jersey. His parents had migrated to the United States of America from Russia.

Henry and Hettie had three children of which Albert was the first. His brother, Paul, was one-and-a-half years younger than him, whereas his sister Janet was four years younger. Ellis' father was a businessman and in 1915, he changed his surname from Groots to Ellis probably to make himself more acceptable in the world of business. As he was on the lookout for better opportunities, he moved his family to New York City when Albert was four years old.

Albert's mother was a good-looking, happy-go-lucky woman. She was fond of socializing with friends, going to parties and enjoying life. She was so busy pursuing her pleasurable activities that she had little time for household work and looking after her husband and children.

Albert's father was a travelling salesman and a promoter and therefore was mostly away from home. Even when he was living with his family, he was engrossed in his business activities.

Since his early childhood, Albert had very good relations with Paul. In fact, no member of his family felt so much affinity towards other members. When Paul was young, he had a tendency to get into trouble. On the contrary, Albert carefully remained away from trouble. Paul was a rebel in his childhood and improved his behaviour in the future and lived a very conventional life. He took a job in the accounts department of a company and worked there until retirement. He almost always followed Albert's teachings. Albert became an unconventional and rebellious adult in the future.

Janet was different from her two brothers. Emotionally dependent on her mother, she was given to whining and crying. This tempted Albert and Paul to get angry with her and to harbour negative thoughts about her. In spite of being the most pampered among the three children, she was afflicted with anxiety, self-hatred and depression. It *should* be noted that only in her 50s did she use REBT to overcome her temperamental handicaps and adopted a healthy and markedly religious way of life.

Albert interpreted the circumstances around him in the very different ways than Janet and Paul. He was a semi-orphan in his childhood. Yet, he managed not to be miserable. He accepted that his life was going to be tough and there was no use of protest against his parents. He decided to use his mind to get along well with his mother as well as his younger siblings and learn to live as happily as possible in the given circumstances. He adjusted to his father's absence and his mother's lack of concern for her children without disturbing himself.

When he was eight years old, he took charge of household activities and carefully planned his daily schedule. He used to get up early in the morning, make and eat his breakfast and get ready to go to school before his mother gets up in the morning. After returning home from school, Albert used to eat some self-prepared snack and feed and look after his younger brother and sister. In this way, he turned the situation to his advantage by developing autonomy and independence.

Parental neglect, however, was not the only handicap in his early life. As a child, he had other problems too. The most troublesome among them was his poor health. He was physically weak as an infant, probably suffered from severe spasmodic abdominal pain and cried a lot. At the age of five, he came down with tonsillitis which developed into a serious strep infection. Emergency surgery saved his life. As a sequel to his surgery, he developed acute nephritis. As a result of this ailment, he was hospitalized eight times between the ages of five and seven. Once, his hospitalization even lasted for 10 months.

His parents rarely visited him at the hospital. In the beginning, he felt angry and depressed. However, he soon realized that the situation was not going to improve and therefore learned to make himself feel quite sorrowful but not very disturbed about his deprivation. That is probably how he discovered that even when the circumstances were not favourable, he could choose the quality and intensity of emotional response. Instead of whining about the unhappy situation, he looked at it as somewhat advantageous. He made friends with children in the hospital and managed to become their leader by inventing a game which they all played.

In his autobiography, Ellis (2010) recalls that even as a child, he realized that he could choose how to react to the parental neglect he was subjected to. That realization proved to be a significant event in his life. He felt that the origin of REBT's concept of healthy and unhealthy emotions lies behind the above realization.

When Albert was hospitalized again and again, his schooling was disrupted. However, he was not unduly bothered about these disruptions. His intelligence quotient, estimated on the basis of his school performance at that time, was between 135 and 160; therefore, it was very easy for him to do outstandingly well in his studies. He could easily overcome the repeated disruptions by skipping two grades in grammar school.

Ellis (2010) said that the first sensible thing he did to help himself enjoy life was to adapt to school as quickly as possible because there was no way to escape the situation. It seems that he was really born with the ability to philosophize and use his head to save himself from parental troubles. Whenever unhappy, he consciously tried to think and find out how he could make himself happy. That is why in an interview with Windy Dryden he said that he was born therapist for himself (Dryden & Ellis, 1989)!

When Albert was six years old, he found a new friend, Manny Birnbaum, who eventually became his best friend, besides, of course, Paul. Soon Albert, Paul and Manny became bosom friends. Their common interests were long walks, visits to the public library and discussions. In addition, they enjoyed playing chess, cards, and watching movies. Nevertheless, Albert, Paul and Manny had really close ties of friendship among themselves in their childhood. They were interested in reading and other intellectual pursuits, and they thought they were unique in comparison to the other children in their neighbourhood.

Among the three of them, Albert probably had a bent for intellectual books. At the tender age of eight or so, he devoured every volume of an encyclopaedia entitled *Book of Knowledge*, which he found in his intellectually impoverished home.

Paul and Manny remained his close friends throughout his life and served on the board of directors of the Albert Ellis Institute. Manny was his personal as well as the Institute's accountant.

Manny, however, might be right in believing that the entire Ellis family were a 'cold bunch' showing very little feelings. That may be the reason why Ellis seemed aloof and cold to many people. It is therefore, not surprising that years later, REBT was criticized for ignoring emotions. However, those who have seen him at close quarters remark that he was a friendly person.

Later Schooldays

A major event happened in Albert's life when he was 12 years old. He overheard a conversation between his mother and his aunt Fanny and realized that his father had divorced his mother about six months ago. His mother had earlier found out that her husband was having an affair with Rose, her best friend. Albert's father was never devoted to his family, even before the divorce. There had never been any strong bond of affection between him and Albert. After their divorce, his mother and father began to live in separate houses. Thereafter, Albert's father rarely visited his wife and children. He did not even give alimony payments to his ex-wife and children on several occasions because of insufficient money. The financial condition of the family was not good and at one time, the three children, now in their early teens, had to start earning money by doing odd jobs such as selling newspapers or matching pants. Albert graduated from the New York High School at the age of 16 and his rank was 17 in the class of about 150 students.

In his high school days, Albert's appetite for reading grew day by day. He gradually lost interest in the popular novels of Frank Merriwell and Horatio Alger. He began to develop a keen interest in political, philosophical and other scholarly books. Along with his formal education, his galloping self-education also enriched his mind and helped him develop some specific political and philosophical views. In addition to reading the works of eminent literary giants, he drank in the writings of the world's great philosophers. At the age of 16, he had studied many philosophers including Epictetus, Spinoza, Kant and Bertrand Russell. Similarly, he read Emerson's renowned essay, Self-reliance, and other self-help books along with books by Sigmund Freud.

When Albert was 12 years old, an event occurred which had a great impact on his life. He read a book on physical geography which shattered his belief in the existence of God. He felt that he was being cheated by religion and its account of creation. He became an atheist. This newly formed rebellious outlook on religion got deeply rooted in his mind. He came to the conclusion that atheism was extremely important for him and for others as well. Since then, he remained an unrepentant atheist.

When he was almost 16, he got acquainted with one boy, named Sid, who was keenly interested in philosophy. Sid drove him into the magnificent world of philosophers. Albert plunged wholeheartedly into philosophy. While reading the works of great philosophers, he also maintained a diary in which he recorded his disagreements with famous philosophers. His interest in philosophy was strong, but he was especially interested in the philosophies which he thought might serve as a source of guidance on how to live life.

It is worth emphasizing that Ellis' interest in philosophy, which manifested itself since his teenage, was one of the most important factors which contributed to the secular and humanistic system of psychotherapy he subsequently created and developed. In his writings, he repeatedly stated that for creating his system of psychotherapy in 1955, he drew considerably on the writings of ancient and modern philosophers rather than on the writings of psychologists and other mental health professionals.

College Education

Albert's passion for reading started to blossom into a dream of becoming a writer. His dream was to become a writer or, to be more specific, a famous novelist. Becoming an accountant and earning a lot of money was the first step in his plan of actualizing his cherished dream. This would give him financial security and the freedom to write anything he chose. Hence, completing high school education, he got admission for BBA degree in the City College of New York, where the residents of New York City were not required to pay tuition fees. As regards the college curriculum, Albert had no difficulty whatsoever. Although he had no liking for accounting, he did well in college just as he had always done in high school. At the age of 20, he obtained a BBA degree in accounting.

During his college life, he did not focus all his time and energy only on studies. He also endeavoured to improve some of the handicapping facets of his personality. In the process, his self-education not only brought about some radical changes in his personality but also helped him develop some concepts which were subsequently merged with his system of psychotherapy.

He was a procrastinator in high school and continued to be so in college. He soon realized that his habit of procrastination was self-defeating; therefore, that habit became the first target of his self-development programme. This programme was later known in his life as the 'Five Minute Plan'.

At the age of 19, he decided to work on his phobia of public speaking. He could speak to people individually and to small circles of friends. This phobia proved to be a major problem for Albert when he began to take active interest in politics by joining Young America and New America, an organization founded by a music teacher and aimed at bringing about America's economic growth. Albert was quite influenced by it, and for about a year, he served as its paid revolutionist. Thus, politics presented a challenge to his rebellious nature and in order to accept that challenge, he made up his mind to get rid of his anxiety of public speaking in the first place. He came up with two concrete steps based on philosophies he read about. They helped him overcome his phobia of public speaking to a large extent. The first step eventually got incorporated in REBT with the descriptive names unconditional self-acceptance (USA) and high frustration tolerance (HFT).

The second step Albert took towards conquering his anxiety about public speaking was to carefully study experiments in conditioning and deconditioning fear responses in children conducted by John B. Watson and R. Rayner (1920). Thus, he became acquainted with the technique of desensitization of fear responses. Encouraged by learning this technique, he began to decondition his phobia about public speaking. He began to give political talks in spite of his anxiety and discomfort. The political organization for which Albert worked as a paid revolutionist did not last long. However, the invaluable lessons he taught himself while working for that organization greatly influenced his later life and work.

Albert's shyness, however, was quite a problem for him. It was also the cause of another severe handicap in his life. Although he wished to date many women, he never dared to directly approach anybody among them. During his adolescence, Albert satisfied his craving for the company of girls by manipulating his male friends to help him get acquainted with women. However, he felt that this method of speaking to girls was perpetuating and strengthening his anxiety. Hence, in the summer of 1933, he arrived at the conclusion that he had better give up his anxiety about approaching women just as he had successfully given up his phobia about public speaking.

To achieve this objective, he gave himself a two-fold homework assignment. Ellis (2010) believed that homework assignment radically changed his own life and, in some respects, the history of psychotherapy as well. As the first part of that two-fold homework assignment, he began to challenge the ideas underlying his anxiety. This technique of disputation acquired a central place in REBT in subsequent years.

Albert's second part of the two-fold assignment to himself consisted of behaving in a new manner by deliberately facing the possibility of getting rejected by women. By implementing this two-fold assignment, he took the risk of talking to 130 women in just about a month. In order to face criticism of others and to increase emotional strength, he even undertook many adventurous experiments which were eventually recognized as 'Shame Attacking Exercises'.

Albert's successful experiments taught him some important lessons which later became a major influence in the creation of his system of psychotherapy. The most important among them was the profound importance of cognition, philosophy, reasoning, and self-persuasion in changing one's dysfunctional feelings and behaviour. In fact, from 1943 to 1947, that is, before learning psychoanalysis, he made the understanding of cognitive processes one of the central features of his technique of psychotherapy. Afterwards, when he gave up practising psychoanalysis upon finding it ineffective and resorted to active-directive therapy in 1953, he stressed the importance of cognition again and again.

Albert's yet another remarkable self-help venture was to release himself from insomnia. Since his early teens, he was afflicted with this malady owing to which he could sleep only a few hours at nights and that too not comfortably. He soon realized that his suffering was caused by two problems. The first problem was insomnia, of course. The second problem was his anxiety about insomnia. He also understood that his second problem, namely, the anxiety about insomnia, was actually interfering with his sleep.

Albert developed his own unique method to cope with the insomnia. His efforts also led him to an important discovery about psychological disturbance in general. His discovery was that a man disturbs himself about some problem in his life at the beginning. Then he disturbs himself about making himself disturbed about that problem. In this way, he creates multiple layers of disturbance. This discovery contained the seed of a major contribution Albert subsequently made to psychotherapy—the concept of disturbance about disturbance.

Unsuccessful Marriage

When Albert earned his BBA degree from City College, the nation was in the grip of the Great Depression. The financial condition of Albert's family was not satisfactory. His mother's savings were completely wiped out. As Albert's father was relatively poor during the Depression, he paid no alimony to Albert's mother. Albert was desperate to get a suitable employment but could not find anything due to scarce job opportunities. He had to continue his old pant matching enterprise, which he started with Paul. However, the income generated from it was so meagre that it was insufficient to meet their daily needs.

Albert even tried to work in a couple of businesses initiated by his father. These collaborative ventures did not produce expected results. In 1938, he began to work as the assistant to the president of a gift and novelty concern called Distinctive Creations. He held that job for almost 10 years, working part-time at the beginning and full-time later.

Albert's struggle to earn his living did not detract him from reading and writing. In the late 1930s and 1940s, he continued to write many novels, plays and poems. As a result, not less than 20 full-length manuscripts of his prolific literary output became available for publishers. However, there were no takers for them.

In 1936, when he was 23 years old, he madly fell in love with a beautiful and vivacious 19-year-old theatre actress named Karyl, but her behaviour towards him was erratic. Sometimes she was warm and friendly but at other times, she would neglect him to a large extent. Moreover, she was indecisive about the plan of marrying him.

One midnight, Albert went to take a walk by the lake in Bronx Botanical Garden to review his shaky affair with Karyl. After pondering over the issue, he realized that he was not troubled by his strong unfulfilled desire for Karyl, rather he was troubled by his unfulfilled dire need for her love. There was nothing awful about not having her love. He not only learned to differentiate between his desires and needs but also to retain his desires and surrender his needs. The two conclusions he drew after pondering over his unstable relationship with Karyl were the prototypes of the two fundamental concepts of his system of psychotherapy. First, human beings become unhappy when they believe that they need (not only want) something. Second, they also suffer when they believe that it is terrible (not only too bad) when they don't get what they think they absolutely need.

On the following day, he met Karyl and told her how he rid himself of his need for her and proposed to her. She was impressed by his newly found philosophy and suggested that they get married in secret since her parents were not happy with his appearance and financial prospects.

Accordingly, in 1938, when Albert was twenty-four, they got married secretly. But that same evening Karyl informed her parents about their marriage. Her parents were furious and forced Albert to proceed for a divorce immediately. Albert agreed to do so because Karyl denied supporting him. However, his relationship with her did not end with the annulment of their marriage.

After a few months, Karyl frantically approached Albert for help in bringing her out from a nervous breakdown that she was suffering from due to the betrayal of her new lover. Without getting emotionally involved with her, Albert helped her wholeheartedly. He encouraged her to establish a healthy relationship with the other man, whom she later married. Albert and Karyl remained friends until she died of emphysema and lung cancer in 2001. Before her death, she often attended Ellis' public therapy sessions and not only acknowledged him as a genius but wished that she had lived with him. If Ellis had been asked about any sadness or regret regarding his unsuccessful marriage, he would have answered in the negative. He would have replied that his biggest learning point from that event was that he was able to review the concept of 'love at first sight'.

The Solo Battle

Albert's unusual relationship with Karyl motivated him to write a revolutionary volume on sex. In spite of his prolonged lack of success in getting any book published, his unflinching determination to write was not at all shaken. With this determination, he went to the New York Public Library. For two years, he read hundreds of books and thousands of articles on sex, love and marriage. Eventually, he did complete the fat volume, *The Case for Sexual Promiscuity*. He sent the manuscript to several publishers but received no affirmative answer from even one of them. In 1965, that is, almost 20 years after the book was written, only its first part was published, bearing the title, *The Case for Sexual Liberty* (Ellis, 1965).

His friends and relatives soon came to know that he was something of a walking encyclopaedia on erotic fiction and non-fiction. They began asking for his advice on tackling some of their problems regarding love and sex. Surprisingly enough, they found his advice useful. He also enjoyed counselling people who were beset with problems. He then seriously reconsidered his dream of becoming a writer. Soon he realized that writing career was not considered as well-paid profession. Hence, he decided to follow the career path indicated by his innate talent for counselling. Consequently, he founded the service called 'Love and Marriage Problems Institute' (LAMP Institute).

His decision to set himself up as a psychological counsellor was not safe enough to implement. In view of his lack of credentials in the area of psychological counselling, his lawyer alerted him to the possibility of legal troubles. Albert accepted the reality, wound up his institute and decided to get professional training in his self-chosen field. He obtained his MA degree in clinical psychology with honours from Teachers College in 1943.

Albert now was a qualified psychologist and began to practise as a counsellor from his residence. Over a period of time, he was able to have three or four clients a week. As a novice in the field of counselling, he was experimenting with different methods and was inclined to adopt more active methods. It took many years for him to find and finally create a system of psychotherapy (i.e., REBT) which was congruent with his temperament and philosophy of life.

While Albert was trying to establish himself as a practising clinical psychologist and continuing his work on Distinctive Creations, he was also pursuing his goal of doing research for his PhD degree on the topic of love and sexual emotions of college women. However, he had to surmount many obstacles that came in his way. Some prudish professors objected to his research topic very strongly. These professors were so adamant and powerful that Albert had to compromise by choosing the distinctly different topic of personality testing for his doctoral research. He acquired his PhD degree in 1947. He could have continued to work in the area of personality testing for the rest of his life, but he chose the path of a practising psychologist.

However, his laboriously acquired knowledge of sex, love relations and marriage in his early career did not go in vain. Later, around 1960, Ellis was one of the founders of the American sexual revolution. He was well known as a liberal sexologist, and he enriched the field of sexology by publishing almost 18 books on the topics of sexuality and love and a number of articles advocating sexual liberation.

Entry into the Profession

Albert was now Dr Albert Ellis, all set to commence his career as a professional psychologist. Now onwards, we will address him with a short and easy title, Ellis.

When Ellis entered the field, psychoanalysis was an established method of psychotherapy. Hence, he began to get himself psychoanalyzed by Dr Charles Hulbeck who was a renowned training analyst. In the next two years, Ellis became a well-trained psychoanalyst.

In 1948, he resigned from Distinctive Creations and took a job as senior clinical psychologist at the Northern New Jersey Mental Hygiene Clinic, which was located at the New Jersey State Hospital in Morristown. This job gave him a good opportunity to interview, test and treat varied types of clients. In addition, in the first year of his service, he wrote not less than 12 research papers. Before him, no state psychologist had published any research papers. He became the blue-eyed boy of the State Department of Institutions and Agencies. As a result, in 1949, he was appointed as chief psychologist of the then newly started New Jersey State Diagnostic Center.

Research papers and books published by Ellis stirred up a hornet's nest. His writings on sex were not very favourably looked upon by Sanford Bates who was the Commissioner of the State Department of Institutions and Agencies. He did not like Ellis' first book called *The Folklore of Sex* (Ellis, 1951). He could not tolerate Ellis' sexual liberalism revealed in that book. With the help of one of his associates, he decided to throw Ellis out of service. Some flimsy charges were levelled against Ellis. Ellis could have defended himself easily and gotten rid of these charges, but he did not do so. The main reason for this was that he did not want to be in service for a long time. As an individualist and rebel, he was not exactly suitable to be in service throughout his life. His plan was to leave the job and devote himself completely to his private practice, research and writing.

In view of these considerations, Ellis left his job in 1952 and thereby threw off the shackles of service. This move was not a response to his entrepreneurial urge. Rather, it was a response to his urge for independence and freedom from censorship.

Emergence of Rational Therapy

Ellis was all set to devote his energies to his private practice on a full-time basis. He adopted psychoanalysis as his main method of counselling. Within a short time, he began to earn enough money to ensure a comfortable life. He saw about 16 clients for 45-minute sessions each day.

However, gradually he developed some misgivings about psychoanalysis. Although it was considered to be a real depth therapy, he came to the conclusion that psychoanalysis was quite ineffective as a system of therapy. Perhaps psychoanalysis did help clients to understand some of the inner psychological causes of their disturbances. However, this insight into their own mental disturbances was not enough to bring about the necessary changes in their thoughts, emotions and behaviours. Naturally, they were unable to overcome their disturbances.

Consequently, Ellis gave up classical psychoanalysis and began to experiment with non-classical, Neo-Freudian psychotherapies. Until 1953, Ellis carefully studied hundreds of other available methods of psychotherapy and tried them out with his clients. None of them could satisfy his urge to improve the effectiveness of psychotherapy. This time, his hobby of reading philosophy came to his rescue and his tireless groping for some effective system of psychotherapy bore fruit. He was convinced that a man's philosophy of life plays an extremely important role in his mental health or mental illness. Of course, he knew the cardinal principle of the Stoic philosophy elaborated by the ancient Greek philosopher Epictetus: 'People are disturbed not by things but by the views they take of them'. This dictum provided him with a key to understand and cure psychological disturbance. As he himself puts it, he 'managed to bring Epictetus out of near-obscurity and make him famous all over again'.

At last in 1954, Ellis started creating a new system of psychotherapy by combining all his psychological and philosophical knowledge. A couple of years prior to this, he had stopped calling himself a psychoanalyst. Instead, he had begun to consider himself a psychotherapist. By that time, he arrived at the conclusion that man's psychological disturbance was created by his irrational, unrealistic and dysfunctional philosophy of life. Finally, in January 1955, Ellis created what he first called rational therapy (RT). Eventually, he hoisted the flag of rebellion by presenting the paper, 'Rational Psychotherapy', at the Annual Convention in Chicago on 31 August 1956.

During this time, few transitions were happening in his personal life too. In 1956, he got married to Rhoda, a young and attractive dancer. However, this marriage did not last long. Within a period of two years, they separated and filed for divorce on mutual agreements. However, without going into bitter memories, Ellis helped her in her time of difficulty. Even after Rhoda's divorce to Ellis, she paid tribute to Ellis in the book *Will the Real Albert Ellis Please Stand Up?* (Di Mattia & Lega, 1990) by saying that Ellis was a psychologist of great genius.

Well-established Psychotherapist

After inventing Rational Therapy in January 1955, Ellis began to use it extensively in his private practice. Struck by the proselytizing bug, he gave many talks and wrote articles on his newborn baby. By the late 1960s, Ellis established himself as a creator, practitioner, trainer and educator of Rational Therapy. In 1955, he found the mission of his life. Since then, he pursued his mission single-mindedly until his last breath. He worked relentlessly to show people that their irrational beliefs are the main cause of their emotional upsets, even when they are beset with adverse circumstances. Adverse circumstances, per se, are not enough to upset them; people had better manage their beliefs towards adverse circumstances in their life.

Ellis's first book on Rational Therapy, *How to Live with a Neurotic: At Home and at Work* (Ellis, 1957) was published in 1957. Since then, Ellis wrote or edited more than 75 books and monographs. He also published more than 800 scientific papers and more than 200 audio and video cassettes. Many of his books had been translated into several languages.

In 1959, Ellis established a non-profit organization called the Institute for Rational Living with the mission to advance and popularize REBT and to train professionals in Rational Therapy in a more formal manner. As days passed, Ellis' Rational Therapy achieved a noteworthy place among the professional therapists. The Institute for Rational Living was accredited as a training institute by the State Board of Regents of New York. In 1964,

Ellis bought a six-storey mansion on 65th Street in Manhattan. He lived there on the top floor. In the next 45 years, this institute not only served as the world's headquarters of REBT but also boasted of having affiliated training centres in the United States of America, Canada, Argentina, Germany, France, England, Romania, Italy, Israel, Australia and others.

However, behind this success, there were a lot of struggles and obstacles. When Ellis began to give talks and write articles and books on Rational Therapy, he had a lot of resistance in the beginning. His critics said that he misunderstood the nature and force of emotions. Classical Freudians also took offense at his critical observations about psychoanalysis. Many therapists felt that Rational Therapy was too intellectual and that it took no cognizance of the emotional aspect of human disturbance.

In reality, from the beginning, Rational Therapy used a wide spectrum of emotional and behavioural aspects of human disturbance. In order to emphasize this fact, in 1961, he changed the name from Rational Therapy to Rational Emotive Therapy (RET). Even then, the critics argued that the behavioural aspect of human disturbance was neglected in RET. In order to correct this misrepresentation, in 1993, he changed the name RET to 'Rational Emotive Behaviour Therapy' (REBT).

In 1965, Ellis began to offer a very novel psycho-educational programme called the Friday Night Workshops. In these workshops, he used to give live demonstrations of rational emotive therapy to volunteers from the audience. In 1966, the institute began a new venture by starting its own journal called *Rational Living*. It had continued to flourish until today, though under revised titles from time to time. In 1971, he founded a school named 'Living School' which was designed to train the children in emotional health and well-being. Apart from these ventures, Ellis contributed many other concepts and techniques to REBT. Today, REBT has been applied to domains other than mental health such as education, politics, philosophy, business, industry, community services, global peace, genetic counselling and many others.

During the last four decades, Ellis had influenced a very large number of psychologists, psychiatrists, psychotherapists and counsellors throughout the world. Professionally, Ellis was an internationally well-established psychologist. He acted in several capacities throughout his life. He was a member of several prestigious psychological institutions and contributed to dozens of scientific journals. Many renowned professional societies offered Ellis their highest professional and clinical awards for his impact on the field of psychology. He was ranked as one of the 'most influential psychologists' by American and Canadian psychologists and counsellors.

As regards Ellis' personal life, it took a significant turn in 1964. He met a tall, slender, attractive and intelligent woman named Janet L. Wolfe. When Ellis met her, he was 51 years old and she was only twenty-four years old. They fell madly in love with each other. After the second divorce, Ellis was not in favour of marrying again. Hence, they entered into a live-in relationship. This unusual relationship lasted for 37 years.

Before coming into contact with Ellis, Janet had a brief work experience in the publishing field. Encouraged by Ellis, she went back to Columbia University and completed her BA in sociology in 1969. Subsequently, she began her graduate education at the New York University and obtained a PhD degree in clinical psychology. She proved to be very efficient office manager of the Ellis' institute as the executive director. During her 37 years at the institute, she made important contributions to its functioning and growth. In 2002, when Ellis was an 88-years-old ailing man, Janet decided to break up the relationship and set up her independent practice. Ellis accepted the grim reality with equanimity and grace and surmounted it bravely.

Final Years

An account of the physical disabilities Ellis developed over years and the way he continued to overcome their debilitating effects to maintain and even enhance his efficiency and productivity will shed considerable light on some facets of his personality.

When Ellis was 19, he was afflicted with renal glycosuria. He found difficulty in reading and therefore began to wear glasses. Perhaps, this was due to renal glycosuria—a precursor of diabetes. Since that age, he suffered from chronically tired eyes and found no remedy for that suffering all his life. He accepted this limitation of his eyes without whining and also learned to live with them. However, even with this handicap, he saw over 80 individuals and about 40 more group clients per week.

At the age of 42, he was diagnosed with type-1 insulin-dependent diabetes. As he grew older, his diabetes continued to handicap his work schedule. Over the years, he had learned that taking 12 small meals a day round the clock kept his blood sugar low, warded off insulin shock reactions and helped maintain a healthy weight. Being a diabetic, he had to face many other health problems too. In his late 60s, Ellis' ability to hear began to reduce and by the time he was in his mid-70s, he started to use two hearing aids. In the final years of his life, he had to take medical help for almost every organ. How Ellis looked at his many physical disabilities throws light upon his attitude towards dealing with the adversities. He viewed them as a challenge to his philosophy of life. The first thing he did in order to cope with his disabilities was to accept them without whining or indulging in self-denigration or self-pity. The second thing he did was to devise ways and means of coping with those disabilities as efficiently as possible. In short, he used his system of psychotherapy to help himself—and he did that brilliantly! When he was 82 years old, he wrote an article describing how he was using his own system of psychotherapy to cope with his disabilities. It not only gave a vivid account of how he used REBT techniques to help him live happily and productively in spite of his disabilities but also explained how he helped his clients cope with their disabilities by applying those techniques.

Despite the series of health issues and profound hearing loss, Ellis typically worked at least 16 hours a day. It is amazing to see his work record of 365 days. In one year's time, he used to conduct 3,015 individual sessions of 30 minutes and 709 sessions of 60 minutes, 62 speeches at various places, 5 group sessions in every week and 9 hours intensive therapy to 12 fellows. The number of books, articles, research papers and reviews he worked on are not even referred in this list.

Ellis' health presented a major challenge to him just a few months before he was 90 years old. He had to undergo a major surgical operation due to severe intestinal problem which led to his hospitalization and the removal of his large intestine. He resumed work almost immediately after being discharged. He was so eager and enthusiastic to continue his mission that on 25 July 2003, he managed to give an as usual workshop on anxiety to the summer fellows. The only difference was in the location. He conducted it in his own bedroom.

Undergoing a major surgical operation at a very advanced age in his life was indeed challenging, but not a mentally shattering experience for Ellis. That unprecedented challenge in his life taught him the realities about the doctors, nurses, and other people who attended to him. Similarly, he learned about the good and bad behaviour of people at his own institute. During this difficult time, Debbie Joffe, a fortyish Australian psychologist and his closest confidante, supported him greatly. When Ellis was in the hospital, she was with him round the clock. The relationship with Debbie became increasingly intimate and culminated in their marriage in 2004. She collaborated with him on writing and research projects thereafter.

By early 2004, when Ellis' health was declining, a bitter feud erupted between Ellis and the board of his own institute over the management policies. He filed a lawsuit against the institute after the board voted him off and cancelled his popular Friday night workshops. Ellis was reinstated to the board in January 2006 after winning civil proceedings against the board members who removed him.

Though the fight saddened Ellis deeply, he reinstated his Friday night workshops in the building next door with the help of Debbie. 'Nothing stopped him', Debbie said. 'Wherever he had an opportunity to contribute, he did, no matter the circumstances'. In April 2006, Ellis was hospitalized with pneumonia and spent more than a year shuttling between hospital and a rehabilitation centre. His extended illness led to kidney and heart failures and he died aged 93 at his residence on 24 July 2007.

During his illness, one journalist asked him, 'Your routine of 16 hours is getting disturbed now. Do you face any difficulty in coping up with this disturbed routine?' Ellis replied promptly, 'Not at all! Now I am able to use these 16 hours in reflection and contemplation!' His reply was true in every sense. Even on the deathbed, he was reforming the REBT theory. The book that contains this reformation was published after his death bearing the title, *Personality Theories: Critical Perspectives* (Ellis, Abrams & Abrams, 2009).

His autobiography entitled *All Out*! (Ellis, 2010) and another book on REBT (Ellis & Ellis, 2011) were published by Debbie in 2010 and 2011 respectively. Throughout his life, Ellis practised what he preached. Hence, one cannot help agreeing with Daniel Wiener (1988) when he says that Ellis's life was his message; they were integral.

'I will retire when I am dead', Ellis said at 90, 'While I am alive, I want to keep doing what I want to do. See People. Give workshops Write and preach the gospel according to St. Albert' (Kaufman, 2007).

In eulogy of Ellis, the past president of APA, Frank Farley (2009), stated,

> Psychology has had only of a handful of legendary figures who not only command attention across much of the discipline but also receive high recognition from the public for their work. Albert Ellis was such a figure, known both inside and outside of psychology for his astounding originality, his provocative ideas, and his provocative personality. He bestrode the practice of psychotherapy like a colossus. (pp. 215–16)

No doubt, Farley's felicitous tribute to Ellis' work captures the significance of his legendary work!

References

Di Mattia, D., & Lega, L. (Eds). (1990). *Will the Real Albert Ellis Please Stand Up? Anecdotes by His Colleagues, Students and Friends Celebrating His 75th Birthday.* New York, NY: Albert Ellis Institute.

Dryden, W., & Ellis, A. (1989). An efficient and passionate life. *Journal of Counseling and Development, 67*(10), 539–46.

Ellis, A. (1951). *The Folklore of Sex.* (Rev. ed., 1961). New York, NY: Grove Press.

———. (1957). *How to Live with a Neurotic: At Home and at Work.* North Hollywood, CA: Wilshire. *How to Live with a Neurotic* (Rev. ed., 1975). New York, NY: Crown.

———. (1965). *The Case for Sexual Liberty.* Tucson, AZ: Seymour Press.

———. (2010). *All Out! Albert Ellis with Debbie Joffe Ellis: An Autobiography.* Amherst, NY: Prometheus Books.

Ellis, A., & Joffe Ellis, D. (2011). *Rational Emotive Behavior Therapy. (Theories of Psychotherapy).* Magination Press, American Psychological Association, United States.

Ellis, A., Abrams, M., & Abrams, L. (2009). *Personality Theories: Critical Perspectives.* Los Angeles, CA: SAGE.

Farley, F. (2009). Albert Ellis (1913–2007). *American Psychologist, 64*(3), 215–16.

Kaufman, M. (2007, July 25). Albert Ellis, 93, Influential Psychotherapist, dies. *The New York Times.* Retrieved from *www.nytimes.com/2007/07/25/nyregion/25ellis.html.*

Watson, J.B., & Rayner, R. (1920). Conditioned Emotional Reactions. *Journal of Experimental Psychology, 3*(1), 1–14.

Wiener, D.N. (1988). *Albert Ellis: Passionate Skeptic.* New York, NY: Praeger.

Further Readings

Ellis, A. (1990). My Life in Clinical Psychology. In C.E. Walker (Ed.), *The History of Clinical Psychology in Autobiography* (pp. 1–37). Homewood, IL: Dorsey.

———. (2004). *REBT: It Works for Me, It Works for You.* Amherst, NY: Prometheus Books.

Epstein, R. (January–February 2001). The prince of reason: An interview with Albert Ellis. *Psychology Today,* 66–76.

Yankura, J., & Dryden, W. (1994). *Albert Ellis.* New Delhi: SAGE.

3

Historical Development of REBT

The birth process of REBT was not smooth. Before its inception, Ellis had many reservations about the efficacy of existing psychotherapies, but none of them had any concrete explanations for his objections. All his attempts to improve them were futile. There was a lot of unrest and skirmishes in his mind for a long period of time. This compelled him to discover a new system of psychotherapy which would overcome all his concerns. His extensive reading on diverse subjects from philosophy to literature, experimentation with his own and other methods and his experience as a psychotherapist were leading him gradually towards his invention.

Rebel Against Psychoanalysis

In 1952, when Ellis started his full-time private practice, he realized that in order to help people live happily with others, it was first necessary to help them live happily and peacefully with themselves. He underwent systematic training in psychoanalysis as it was the most prevalent method those days. As a trained practitioner of psychoanalysis, Ellis rendered good services to his clients. His therapeutic results were never less effective than the results of other analysts in New York. In fact, about 60 per cent of his neurotic clients improved considerably after undergoing psychoanalysis. It meant that his effectiveness as an analyst was better than the effectiveness of the average analysts in New York. Usually, his clients continued to remain in treatment for a long period of time instead of dropping out of treatment just after their analysis started and even referred their friends and relatives to Ellis.

Yet, he was unhappy with his own effectiveness because he felt that something was missing in the theory and practice of psychoanalysis. For example, he realized that many clients had difficulty in learning the technique of free association. Interpreting the dreams of his clients was by no means an easy task because some clients rarely dreamed and when they did, they forgot their dreams in no time. Some clients could not be on the sofa for a long time. They even jumped up and down in Ellis' office and did not hesitate to tell him that he was not helping them at all.

Apart from these difficulties, Ellis faced a major problem while analysing his clients. Many of them, even after developing a good insight into the deep rooted unconscious causes of their disturbance, did not show any improvement in their present anxieties, hostilities, feelings of inferiority, depression, guilt, inertia and inactivity. Ellis meticulously interpreted his clients' free associates and dreams and showed the causal connection between their past memories and present problems. His clients reported that they were feeling better after being psychoanalyzed, but complained that their handicapped behaviour showed no improvement. Maybe undergoing psychoanalysis helped them understand how they got disturbed, but that understanding provided them with no means of overthrowing their disturbance and reconstructing their personality.

Let's illustrate this point with the case example presented in Case 3.1.

Case 3.1

Case of Joseph

> Imagine that Joseph approached Ellis for anger management. He was throwing anger tantrums at his boss or wife quite often. During psychoanalysis, Ellis convinced him that his current anger was not caused by the nasty behaviour of his wife or boss, but was really caused by the hatred he felt for his father or mother. By getting angry at his boss or wife, he was unconsciously getting back at his father or his mother. Ellis noticed that even after knowing this cause, Joseph did not show any improvement.

Joseph's case made Ellis ponder over this issue. He could not console himself by believing that although his clients developed significant insights into the causes of their disturbance, they still did not really see the relationship between their deeply buried unconscious mental processes and their present handicapping emotions and behaviour. As a result, he gradually became more and more sceptical about the psychoanalysis theory and practice.

Ellis began to consolidate his criticism of psychoanalysis. His central arguments against psychoanalysis can be summarized under three heads. First, the traditional psychoanalysts laid unwarranted emphasis on insight while helping the client overcome his anxieties and hostilities. In reality, the client requires to be persuaded to undertake and execute some plan of action that it designed to combat his anxieties and hostilities. Second, psychoanalysts take a very passive role while helping their clients. Instead, he took a more active and directive role. Last, his methods of interpreting the clients' response were unscientific. Being a rebel, Ellis started voicing his criticism of psychoanalysis by giving lectures and writing articles. Since he still wanted to practise as a psychoanalyst, he tried to reform the system of psychoanalysis from within.

His first critical article on psychoanalysis was published in 1949. Titled 'Towards the Improvement of Psychoanalytic Research' (Ellis, 1949), it outlined four ways of improving psychoanalysis: (a) train the analysts in the scientific method, (b) set higher standards for publishing research, (c) review each other's research more critically and (d) endeavour to rigorously adhere to the scientific approach and method. In 1950, he once again tried to reform psychoanalysis by publishing a monograph titled *An Introduction to the Principles of Scientific Psychoanalysis* (Ellis, 1950), but professional psychoanalysis did not bother to take his well-intentioned criticism of psychoanalysis seriously.

He was convinced that not only was the classical psychoanalytic technique of helping his clients time-consuming but also ineffective. Therefore, he started using neoclassical Non-Freudian techniques of therapy, keeping in mind that liberal psychoanalysis was 'deeper', 'more intensive' and therefore 'more curative'. He tried different models offered by neo-Freudians such as Sandor Ferenczi, Earnest Jones, Otto Fenichel, Erich Fromm, Karen Horney and others.

In short, he began to experiment with psychoanalytically oriented psychotherapy. This kind of psychotherapy was superficial in the sense that it deemphasized the methods of free association and dream analysis, but it permitted him to adopt a more active and quickly interpretative therapeutic method. He found that this adaptation of the classical psychoanalysis method was more efficient and effective.

When Ellis adopted psychoanalytically oriented shorter methods of therapy, his clients improved considerably. Nevertheless, his search for better methods of therapy did not come to an end. It led him to an important question: How did he treat his clients in LAMP having marital and sex problems before he turned to psychoanalysis? The answer was that he used active-directive methods to help his clients overcome their disturbances. In fact, he taught them relevant skills for coping with their practical problems and even gave them homework assignments. These methods were yielding good results. Hence, he incorporated some active directive methods in his psychoanalytically oriented practice of psychotherapy.

From 1950 to 1955, he practised as an active, although still psycho-analytically oriented, psychotherapist. His dissatisfaction with his performance, though reduced to a large extent, was not completely over. Many of his clients did not show the expected improvement in their emotions and behaviour. This was evident in the case of one of his female clients. Let's call her Lucy. Her case is illustrated in Case 3.2.

Case 3.2

Case of Lucy

Lucy had severe anxiety. She refused to approach unknown males in spite of the fact that she was very keen to marry. Psychotherapy certainly helped her see that her parents and relatives had practically taught her to be afraid of strangers. She realized that she was mortally afraid of rejection as she was made to believe that, unlike her younger sister, she was not at all attractive. Further, she gained deep insight into her tremendous fear of shouldering the responsibilities of marriage.

Finally, she fully accepted that she was too attached to her father and did not want to leave him and undertake the risky venture of marriage. Yet, she did nothing to try meeting unknown males although her inaction in this respect was defeating her own goal of marriage.

Like Lucy, Ellis repeatedly came across clients who did not surrender their self-defeating emotions and behaviour and adopt useful emotional and behavioural strategies to achieve their self-chosen goals in spite of developing dramatic insights into the origins of their problems. Gradually, he became disillusioned with the effectiveness of the traditional concept of insight. This compelled him to think about psychotherapy more critically. In the case of Lucy, perhaps her parents and relatives did make her fearful of rejection and of the onerous responsibilities of married life. But who was responsible for the continuation of those fears in her adult life? What explained why her fearful withdrawal from males was not 'extinguished' (in accordance with the Pavlovian theory of conditioning) when it was defeating her own goal of marriage? Was not the non-attainment of her own goal penalizing enough?

Past Observations

In the course of his critical rethinking of the effectiveness of psychotherapy, Ellis began to ponder over how he had overcome his own anxiety of approaching women when he was a shy young man in his early 20s.

This was how he developed his own method to overcome his anxiety about approaching women. Since the age of 16, he had read many articles and books on psychology, self-help and philosophy. He had managed to make himself less unhappy about some of his other problems such as his anxiety about masturbation and procrastination. In those projects, aimed at self-improvement, he had derived more help from the writings of philosophers, novelists, essayists, dramatists, and poets than the writings of psychologists. The writings of Confucius, Gautam Buddha, Epicurus, Epictetus, Marcus Aurelius and other ancient philosopher had profoundly influenced him. Similarly, he had helped himself by reading Western philosophers such as Spinoza, Kant, Hume, Emerson, Thoreau, Santayana.

The central message that he had gleaned from his voracious reading was that human beings largely create their needless misery by irrational and dysfunctional thinking and they can change their thinking and recreate emotional and behavioural fulfilment. Fortunately, this insight into man's emotional upsets had earlier helped him overcome his anxiety about public speaking. Now he was ready to overcome his anxiety about approaching women. Here, it may be recalled that in order to overcome his anxiety about getting rejected by women, he had given himself a two-fold homework assignment. As per his first homework assignment, based on his understanding of human unhappiness, he found out and challenged the beliefs and philosophies underlying his anxiety. This helped him convince himself that even his frequent poor performance in approaching women was not going to prove that he was a *failure*. It would only prove that he was a person who failed many times.

His second homework assignment was based on his knowledge that John B. Watson, the father of behaviourism, and R. Rayner (Watson & Rayner, 1920) had helped young children overcome their fear of mice and rabbits by exposing them to fearful animals. In essence, the techniques of Watson and Rayner consisted of placing the terrifying animals 10 feet away from those children and then gradually bringing the animals close to them. While adopting this procedure, Watson distracted the children by talking to them. The result of this experiment was that in a short period of time, the children gave up their fear and began to pet the same animals. This deconditioning procedure is called '*in vivo* (live) desensitization'. It formed the basis of the second homework assignment that Ellis gave to himself. It consisted of forcing himself again and again to approach female strangers and get rejected many times. This action-oriented assignment finally convinced him that even if he was rejected by women, he was not worthless; although, it was very bad that he was not accepted by some women.

New Insights

This recollection and reconsideration of his personal experience of overcoming his shyness (and also his experience of getting rid of his phobia of public speaking) convinced him that human beings were very unlikely to change their self-defeating behaviour merely by using their ability to think. They would change their behaviour if their thinking was followed by suitable actions. In fact, when he was practising as a professional marriage, family and sex therapist prior to becoming a psychoanalyst, he used to give behavioural homework assignment to clients. He came to the firm conclusion that human beings could get rid of their handicapping emotions and behaviour by changing their thoughts and their actions.

He now could clearly see why psychoanalysis was ineffective. The psychoanalyst helps his clients to gain insight into their mental disturbance by relating that disturbance to some events in their past, but has practically nothing to say about how his clients continue to maintain their disturbances. He also fails to explain to his clients what they did in their past to make themselves mentally disturbed in the first place. Nor can he explain to them why they continue to disturb themselves mentally. The psychoanalyst speaks as if his clients are helpless victims of their past lives. Consequently, not only is his analysis ineffective but it often unknowingly encourages them to pity and even re-traumatize themselves by brooding over the unfortunate events in their past.

Ellis also studied psychotherapy based on the conditioned response theory of Pavlov. He found this approach to human disturbance quite meaningful. Perhaps, in their childhood, humans were conditioned to emote and behave dysfunctionally, therefore they could be treated by following the deconditioning technique invented by Pavlov, but he soon realized its limitations too. The Pavlovian approach suggests that clients are conditioned to feel and behave dysfunctionally because events in their past conditioned them to feel and behave dysfunctionally. This approach seems to assume that clients do not play any active role in bringing about and maintaining their mental disturbance. They are just helpless victims of the events in their past.

Ellis rebelled against both the approaches to psychotherapy—the psychoanalytic approach and the Pavlovian approach. The foundation of his rebellion was his assertion that unlike other animals, human beings are gifted with the capacity to think, to think about what they think and to think about what they think about what they think and so on. Therefore, no matter the traumatizing events that occurred in their lives, they add some of their own thinking to those traumatizing experiences and thereby create mental disturbances. Similarly, they actively contribute to the continuation of their mental disturbance and their contribution is in the form of their ideas, beliefs, attitudes and philosophies of life.

Obviously, the major drawback in a psychoanalyst is that he spends a lot of time unearthing the irrelevant historical data about his clients but rarely focuses on their current ideas, beliefs attitudes and philosophies of life. Moreover, he does not push his clients to act against their handicapping emotions and behaviour. On the contrary, the therapist who follows the Pavlovian theory of conditioned response helps his clients to act against their handicapping emotions and behaviour, but pays no attention to his clients' ideas, beliefs, attitudes and philosophies of life.

The Last Straw

Ellis was disillusioned with psychoanalysis once he clearly understood its major shortcomings. His disillusionment was further aggravated by another important event. In 1953, he did a considerable amount of research for a monograph and a lengthy article on the new techniques in psychotherapy. He studied 431 articles on psychotherapy published since the early 1950s and arrived at some important revelations about what different psychotherapists were doing after they distanced themselves from the psychoanalytic techniques. They began to use the techniques designed to help their client feel better. They did not care whether their techniques were endorsed by the prevailing orthodox theories. Hence, their techniques allowed them to actively help their clients, direct them to set meaningful goals and values and encourage them to focus on the current problems instead of concentrating on the earlier causes of their problems.

Besides, the therapists used different techniques for different people. Also, they felt free to switch from one technique to another depending on the type of client as well as their way of responding to different techniques. Hence, they knew that no single technique worked with most of clients most of the time. These findings led Ellis further away from psychoanalysis. Two years later, in 1955, these findings of his research were published in the form of a monograph titled *New Approaches to Psychotherapy Techniques* (Ellis, 1955).

In 1954, Ellis openly refused to call himself a psychoanalyst. As an uncompromising rebel, he made no secret of the fact that he was against psychoanalysis. Of course, he was determined to formulate and nurture his cognitive primacy theory of emotional disturbance on the basis of his own research and personal experience as a psychotherapist. Although his sincere appeal to reform psychoanalysis went almost unheeded in New York, it did strike a chord in the hearts of some scholars in Minnesota. In 1954, he was invited to present a paper at the conference on Psychoanalysis and Philosophy of Science at the Centre for the Philosophy of Science at the University of Minnesota. This paper (1956) entitled,' An Operational Reformulation of Some of the Basic Principles of Psychoanalysis', was a devastating attack on the traditional and unscientific methods of psychoanalysis, but it made a great impact on the learned members of the audience. He found a kindred spirit in Starke Hathaway who was the leader of clinical psychology at the University of Minnesota. He was teaching and practising down-to-earth, straightforward, no-nonsense methods of doing therapy and his unorthodox approach to therapy was already well established in Minnesota. This scholarly paper of Ellis was published in the journal *Psychoanalytic Review* in 1956.

The Conception of REBT

What was the outcome of Ellis' years of struggle to improve his own effectiveness as a psychotherapist? The main outcome was his profound realization that as human beings, unlike Pavlovian dogs, were capable of thinking and thinking about their thinking, the therapeutic methods based on the Pavlovian concepts of conditioning and deconditioning were not enough to understand and treat human psychological disturbance. He was also convinced that psychoanalysis dealt with irrelevant information about the clients' childhood but failed to pay any serious attention to their current philosophic outlook. He carefully investigated the philosophical or attitudinal basis of human disturbance.

Since the age of 16, he had studied philosophy, especially the philosophy of happiness, as a hobby. Now he returned to the study of philosophy with a specific purpose. He wanted to know how the wisdom of philosophers could be used to help people tackle their emotional problems. Therefore, he began to focus more on the ideas, beliefs, attitudes and philosophies of life of his clients with an objective of understanding and uprooting their emotional and behavioural disturbance. Of course, he gave them in vivo desensitization assignments too. In this way, he welded his therapeutic approach stressing on man's capacity to think with the techniques used in behavioural therapy.

However, as he continued to use more active-directive and elective techniques for helping his clients, he became more and more convinced that human beings were not disturbed by the happenings in their lives but by the meanings they gave to those happenings. These meanings were determined by their ideas, beliefs, attitudes and philosophies of life.

Since 1953, Ellis was actively and rigorously working on his new system of psychotherapy. By the beginning of 1955, the basic theory and practice of what Ellis at that time called 'Rational Therapy' (RT) was so clearly formulated in his mind, that he succinctly propounded it in the philosophy of the ancient Greek philosopher, Epictetus.

Underlying Premises of REBT

In 1955, when Ellis presented RT, it emphasized two salient features: (a) it focused on the client's irrational thinking which he deemed to be at the core of psychological disturbances and (b) the major task of rational therapists was to help clients think rationally about themselves, other people and the world (Dryden, 1990). In the later period, Ellis made several important revisions to REBT from time to time, but the basic premise remained same that events do not directly cause an emotional disturbance. Rather, it is one's beliefs about the events which cause dysfunctional emotions and self-defeating behaviour. REBT teaches clients to identify, evaluate and dispute their irrational self-defeating beliefs, thus helping them not only feel better but get better as well.

However, the role of irrational beliefs in emotional disturbance was not highlighted first by Ellis. He repeatedly pointed out that for formulating his theory of the causes and treatment of emotional disturbance, he heavily borrowed from the writings of both ancient and modern philosophers. Similarly, he concluded that many prominent figures in the field of psychological treatment such as Pierre Janet, Paul Dubois, Alfred Adler and others had propounded cognitive conceptions of psychotherapy in the early twentieth century. However, in the 1950s, their influence had been lessened because of the popularity of the Freudian and to some extent Pavlovian concepts. As a result, when Ellis began to emphasize irrational beliefs as the cause of mental disturbance, he was not readily accepted by the establishment.

How Ellis established and promoted REBT, how it helped him to deal with his clients more effectively, the therapeutic techniques he developed over the period and the insights he stressed on in the therapeutic session will be seen in subsequent chapters.

References

Dryden, W. (1990). *The Essential Albert Ellis. Seminal Writings on Psychotherapy.* New York, NY: Springer Publishing Company.

Ellis, A. (1949). Towards the improvement of psychoanalytic research, *Psychoanalytic Review, 36,* 123–43.

———. (1950). An introduction to the principles of scientific psychoanalysis. *Genetic Psychology Monographs, 41,* 147–212.

———. (1955). New approaches to psychotherapy techniques. *Journal of Clinical Psychology Monograph Supplement, 11,* 1–53.

———. (1956). An operational reformulation of some of the basic principles of psychoanalysis. *Psychoanalytic Review,* 43 (1), 163–180.

Watson, J. B, & Rayner, R. (1920). Conditioned emotional reactions. *Journal of Experimental Psychology, 3*(1), 1–14.

Further Readings

Ellis, A. (1983). The origin of rational-emotive therapy (RET). *Voices: The Art and Science of Psychotherapy, 18*(4), 29–33.

———. (1995). *Better, Deeper and More Enduring Brief Therapy: The Rational Emotive Behavior Therapy Approach* (1st edition). New York: Routledge.

———. (1997). The evolution of Albert Ellis and rational emotive behavior therapy. In J.K. Zeig (Ed.), *The Evolution of Psychotherapy: The Third Conference* (pp. 69–82). New York, NY: Brunner/Mazel.

4
Overview of REBT Theory

'Though I have invented REBT, people give me more credit than I deserve', Ellis once admitted. Moreover, he stated humorously that he had actually stolen the basic premises and theories from ancient philosophers such as Epictetus and Marcus Aurelius. Further, he added, 'If somebody tries to invent an entirely new system of psychotherapy, some of its tenets can be traced somewhere in the history!'

Though Ellis confessed truthfully, no one *should* forget that his confession reveals not only his honesty but his modesty as well. He relentlessly worked towards the development of REBT for more than six decades. He not only expanded the theory but also added many techniques and displayed its application to almost every single area of life. In order to understand the permeation of REBT, we need to review the broad outline of its theory and the changes occurred in it during the past six decades.

The Origin of Emotional Disturbance

The common notion is that events or people around us cause our unhappiness or happiness. Hence, if somebody insults us, we get angry or we feel nervous if we do not get expected appreciation form others. Poor social or economic conditions lead to depression and good music uplifts our mood and reduces our anxiety.

If we review these comments carefully, we will understand that our happiness, unhappiness, joys and misery do not depend only on events or people around us. If outside situation or people cause our misery, then all the people who undergo the same situation or face same people *should* have developed the same emotion. But this is not the reality. If a hundred people are insulted in the same manner, not all of them will get angry. Some of them will remain calm, some will blame themselves, some of them will get anxious and some of them will become hostile. Similarly, the same poor social or economic conditions do not lead to depression in all the people. Not all of them do feel nervous in the case of lack of appreciation and the same music does not uplift their moods or reduce their anxiety. It is evident from the description that more than outside events or people, the meaning that we give to them determine our emotions.

Though this concept is simple, our everyday language is filled up with examples antagonistic to it. How often do we say or hear phrases such as, 'He made me so mad!' Or 'It has got me so upset!' More correctly, we could say, 'I made myself mad' and 'I got myself upset'. How strange would these sound to our ears! Yet the common ingredient in the corrected statements implies an important concept: We are responsible for our emotions. Thus, emotions are not foisted upon us or injected magically into us, but result from something we actively do (Walen, DiGiuseppe & Wessler, 1980).

The following example from *A Practitioner's Guide to REBT* (Walen, DiGiuseppe & Wessler, 1980) may elaborate this point:

> Suppose you are driving and you come across a red light. Does this make you stop? If red lights make you stop, you would brake at all red lights, not just those in traffic signals. If all red traffic lights made you stop, no one would ever go through them or get traffic tickets for doing so. Do you always stop when you come to a red traffic light? No. Not always. Perhaps it is the wee hours of the morning and the streets are deserted. Perhaps you are in a great hurry. Perhaps you are driving to the hospital with your wife, whose labor pains are two minutes apart. In other words, red lights do not always make us behave in a predictable fashion. Other factors can intervene, and these are our attitudes or cognitions about the event the way we interpret it. (p. 15)

The ABC Framework

When REBT was originally established, Ellis had conceived a simple conceptual model to address client's psychological disturbance. This model is known as The ABC framework. In this framework, 'A' stands for *activating event*, which is usually some adverse environmental occurrence. 'B', which is the most important one, is the person's *belief system*. The belief system consists of the meanings, interpretations and evaluations about 'A'. The letter 'C' stands for emotional and behavioural *consequences* or *consequences* to holding the particular *beliefs* at 'B'.

Although different REBT therapists use different versions of the ABC framework, we will stick to the original framework and try to understand it with the help of example in real life situation.

Suppose we find out that our close friend had passed some nasty comments on our behaviour. Let the friend's comments will be 'A'. Our emotions such as anger, insult, hatred and sadness will be 'C'. We commonly believe that the cause of 'C' is 'A'. However, the ABC framework states that the real cause of 'C' is 'B', not A.'

When we come to know our friend's comments, we say to ourselves, 'How ill- natured he is! How cheap is he! He claims to be my closest friend and talks trash when my back is turned! What a betrayal!' These thoughts flash in our mind in less than a few seconds. We get lost in seething rage because of these thoughts. We get encompassed by the emotions of anger, insult, hatred, sadness and many others. We evaluate our friend's behaviour as bad, untrue and ungrateful. This occurs at 'B'. This evaluation leads to emotional upset. Hence, it is not 'A' but 'B' that is the true reason of 'C'.

The ABC framework is followed by 'D', which stands for *disputing* the beliefs that create self-defeating emotional and behavioural consequences (C). For instance, at D, we can vigorously and persistently ask ourselves the following questions: Is there any rule why he *should* not do so? Where has been written that the close friend *should* not pass nasty comments? Just because he once passed nasty comments on my behaviour, does he become totally bad and ungrateful? Were the comments really nasty or just unlikable? Is it not the exaggeration to call unlikable comments as nasty?

As a result of asking these questions repeatedly to ourselves, we realize that our belief (B) regarding labelling other's behaviour on the basis of one instance is irrational. We will begin to accept more rational and realistic beliefs, such as, 'It would be better if he has not done so, but there is no evidence to say that he *should* have not done so. Just because he once passed nasty comments on my behaviour, he does not become totally bad or ungrateful. By labelling his behaviour as nasty, I am exaggerating the severity of the situation and creating disturbing emotions in my mind'.

In this way, when the needless and harmful emotional turmoil in our mind subsides, we will move onto the last letter of this framework, that is, 'E', which represents the development of *effective attitude or philosophy of life*. With the help of ABC framework, how can we solve our emotional problems is more clearly understandable from Figure 4.1.

Figure 4.1

A Method of Solving Emotional Problems

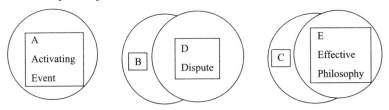

Source: Phadke and Khear (2001).

Thought and Emotions

In the previous example, we have seen how we create most of our feelings by our thinking and how we need to detect and modify the cognitions that underlie them in order to change our emotions. It shows that there is a close relationship between our thoughts and emotions.

Emotion, the main concern of psychotherapy, normally arises from direct stimulation of the cells in hypothalamus and autonomic nervous system. This stimulation can be affected by electrical or chemical agents. It can also be affected indirectly via sensory motor, cognitive and other activity-centred processes.

Naturally, if one is experiencing a very strong emotional upset, he can calm himself down by using one or more of the four available methods:

1. Take electroshock or drug treatment
2. Use soothing baths or relaxation techniques
3. Seek the company of a beloved person and quiet down for his sake or
4. Reason oneself into a state of calmness by showing oneself how irrational it is to remain strongly upset

Although, all the four methods of reducing one's emotional disturbance are legitimate and effective, REBT concentrates on the fourth one, that is, the rational techniques. However, it is necessary to bear in mind that thinking, feeling and behaving are not disparate but are integrally interrelated and are never seen wholly separate from each other. Similarly, thinking and emoting are not two completely different processes. Instead, they very much overlap in many aspects. Further, thinking causes emotion and vice versa. In fact, these processes are so interrelated that they can be considered as one process for all practical purposes.

Although REBT uses the thinking–feeling–acting form of psychotherapeutic treatment, it gives more emphasis on the thinking part. A few of the important reasons of its heavy emphasis on cognition are mentioned here.

1. Human beings have a distinctive capacity to think that differentiates them from other animals. Ellis (1979) says that human beings not only think of complex ways but also have a unique capacity to think about their thinking and, at times, to think about thinking about their thinking.
2. Cognitions (beliefs) can be identified and are easily accessible as compared to emotional and behavioural changes.
3. Changes in only feeling or acting or both may not lead to a significant or long-term improvement. Even if these changes occur, they may be short term in nature. Changes in cognition (core irrational beliefs) often lead to long-term or significant changes.
4. Changes in cognitions (core irrational beliefs) lead to profound philosophical change which are not limited to a specific or the current symptom, but it generalizes to other areas of life which help the client improve his mental health significantly.

REBT therefore is considered as a highly depth-centred and philosophically oriented system of personality change (Ellis, 1968, 1974; Ellis & Grieger, 1977).

Thoughts and Language

We have seen the close ties our thoughts have with our emotions. Now let us see what we actually do when we think. As we can create signs, symbols and languages, our thinking takes the form of the sentences we tell ourselves, that is, our self-talk. As a result, our self-talk becomes our thoughts. These thoughts lead to emotions. This does not mean that emotions cannot exist without thoughts. However, sustained emotions can rarely exist without conscious or unconscious thoughts.

Imagine that one person is going for the job interview and he has following self-talk in his mind:

How many candidates will be there? What would be their qualifications and experience? How would we impress the interviewers? Will they select me or not? Whatever it may be, I will try to give my best! I have prepared well and have related experience too. I think I can impress the interviewers. Even if they do not select me, I will not be devastated. I will learn something from that experience!

If a person has this above self-talk, he will feel hope, confidence, and determined.

Imagine that if he has contrasting self-talk like,

Oh My God! At least 50–60 candidates will be screened. Many will be more educated and experienced than me. How will I get selected among them? What will happen if the interviewers ask me tough questions? What will other people think if I do not get selected? Let's not go for this interview and avoid the stress!

This self-talk leads to hopelessness, fear, anxiety and diffidence in his mind. In nutshell, our self-talk lays at the root of our emotions. This self-talk creates and sustains emotional disturbance, if it is irrational.

REBT assumes that emotional disturbance is caused and maintained by illogical, unrealistic, irrational and illogical thinking. A major corollary of this assumption is that human beings can live the most self-fulfilling, creative and essentially satisfying lives by organizing and disciplining their thinking. That is precisely what an REBT practitioner helps his clients learn and practice. It is necessary to stress on how Ellis explicitly underlined that profound importance of cognition in the creation and treatment of psychological disturbance at the time when therapists were harping on the feelings, feelings, and feelings.

Sustenance of Emotional Disturbance

Let's take one more example. If somebody stamps on our feet, we get furious instantly. Our fury sustains for a long period of time even after the pain in the leg ceases. The reason of this sustenance is the self-talk behind the fury. It would be like, 'How irresponsible are these people! Do not bother about others at all! They do not even have the basic courtesy to say sorry! This is very rude!' It is clear now that whatever the cause of our disturbance, we sustain it by continuing our self-talk for longer periods of time.

This is a significant point in REBT. Ellis says that if we assume that the cause of our present disturbance is in the past incidents, it doesn't answer the question: How do we maintain our disturbance? REBT has the specific answer to this question, that is, if the man is disturbed presently about a past incident, he talks to himself continuously about that incident. Hence, it is not the incident but his self-talk about that incident that maintains his disturbance.

Irrational and Illogical Thoughts

Unfortunately, we examine our self-talk vary rarely. We never bother to check the logical and factual basis of these thoughts. For example, we often talk to ourselves, 'If I fail in the exam or if I do not get selected in the interview or if I disappoint my girlfriend or if I am not become successful in the work, etc.' But we do not examine our self-talk by asking the questions to ourselves that even if these things happen, what disaster is going to befall me? Would it be the end of the world? Will sky fall down on me? If we examine our thoughts on factual ground, we can eradicate our anxiety and fear. There are irrational and illogical thoughts behind every emotional disturbance. Ellis said that if we uproot these irrational thoughts and replace them with rational thoughts, we will be able to reduce our disturbance to a great extent.

Twelve Generic Irrational Beliefs

We need to think more about 'B'. How do we interpret and evaluate the situation around us and behaviour of others? We do it as per our belief systems. This belief system consists of the beliefs towards ourselves, beliefs towards others and beliefs towards the world. These beliefs play an important role in generating our emotions.

Ellis had observed thousands of clients with emotional disturbance in the long tenure of his practice. While treating them, he was convinced that their disturbance was the result of their irrational and illogical beliefs. They were beset by such a maelstrom of these beliefs that their mental health was at risk. Ellis investigated the beliefs held widely by lay people which cause emotional disturbance. He classified them and presented a list of 12 generic irrational beliefs (Ellis, 1994). This list is displayed in Table 4.1. In this list, irrational beliefs are presented on the left side and corresponding rational alternatives are shown on the right side.

Table 4.1

Irrational and Rational Beliefs

No.	Irrational Beliefs	Rational Beliefs
1.	It is a dire necessity for an adult to be loved by everyone for everything he does.	It is better to concentrate on one's own self-respect, on winning the approval of others for practical purposes (such as job advancement) and on loving rather than on being loved.
2.	Certain acts are wrong, or wicked, or villainous, and therefore people who perform such acts *should* be severely punished.	Certain acts are inappropriate or antisocial, and that people who perform such acts are invariably stupid, ignorant or emotionally disturbed.
3.	It is terrible, horrible, and catastrophic when things are not the way one would like them to be.	It is too bad when things are not the way one would like them to be, and one *should* certainly try to change or control conditions so that they become more satisfactory, but that if changing or controlling uncomfortable situations is impossible, one had better become resigned to their existence and stop telling oneself how awful they are.
4.	Much human unhappiness is externally caused and is forced on one by outside people and events.	Virtually all human unhappiness is caused or sustained by the view one takes of things rather than the things themselves.
5.	If something is or may be dangerous or fearsome, one *should* be terribly concerned about it.	If something is or may be dangerous or fearsome, one *should* frankly face it and try to render it non-dangerous and when that is impossible, think of other things and stop telling oneself what a terrible situation one is or may be in.
6.	It is easier to avoid than to face life difficulties and self- responsibilities.	The so-called easy way is invariably the much harder way in the long-run and the only way to solve difficult problems is to face them squarely.
7.	One needs something other or stronger or greater than oneself on which to rely.	It is usually better to stand on one's own feet and gain faith in oneself and one's ability to meet difficult circumstances of living.
8.	One *should* be thoroughly competent, adequate, intelligent and achieving in all possible respects.	One *should* do rather than always try to do well, and one *should* accept oneself as quite an imperfect creature who has general human limitations and specific fallibilities.
9.	Just because something once strongly affected one's life, it *should* indefinitely affect it.	One *should* learn from one's own experiences but not be overly attached to or prejudiced by them.

(Table 4.1 Continued)

(Table 4.1 Continued)

No.	Irrational Beliefs	Rational Beliefs
10.	It is vitally important to our existence what other people do and that we *should* make great efforts to change them in the direction we would like them to be.	Other people's deficiencies are largely their problems and putting pressure on them to change is usually least likely to help them do so.
11.	Human happiness can be achieved by inertia and inaction.	Humans tend to be happiest when they are actively and vitally absorbed in creative pursuits or when they are devoting themselves to people or projects outside themselves.
12.	One has virtually no control over one's own emotions and that one cannot help feeling certain things.	One has enormous control over one's emotions if one chooses to work at controlling them and to practise saying the right kind of sentences to oneself.

Source: Ellis (1994).

Granted that the beliefs[1] (mentioned in Table 4.1) are called irrational on the basis of justifiable grounds, how are people affected by adhering to them? Obviously, such people are likely to become inhibited, hostile, defensive, guilty, ineffective, inert, uncontrolled or unhappy. However, if they throw off these irrational ideas, it would be very unlikely that they will become victims of severe emotional disturbance at least for a very long period.

Four Vital Stages

Now that we know about the commonly held irrational beliefs and their impact, our next focus *should* be on getting rid of them. REBT uses rational analysis and reconstruction to deal with this question. The basic proposition of this model is that the rational, factual and logical thinking improves our mental health. Therefore, the main focus of REBT is on changing the client's faulty thinking. Though the therapeutic process

---

[1] If you want to check the extent to which you hold these beliefs, go to *https://liberomagazine. com/wp-content/uploads/2011/05/Beliefs-Inventory.pdf* and find out your score on each irrational belief.

is described in Chapter 8 in detail, we will quickly review four vital therapeutic stages involved in REBT.

1. To identify the correct self-talk behind the client's dysfunctional emotions
2. To identify the core irrational beliefs manifested by the self-talk
3. To rigorously dispute these irrational beliefs
4. To replace these irrational beliefs with rational beliefs

Case 4.1 will throw more light on the mentioned stages.

Case 4.1

Case of Mr Khanna

Mr Khanna was considered a problem employee in his department because of his resentful attitude towards others and frequent outbursts of anger. His uncontrolled temper was not only adversely affecting his work but also was creating many unnecessary conflicts with others. When he met the therapist, he reported having quarrelled with the clerk in the accounts department. The clerk refused to reimburse Mr Khanna's taxi fare because he was short of cash. Mr Khanna argued with him, shouted at him and lost his temper. He was disturbed and met the therapist.

We will now check how these stages can be implemented in this case. Box 4.1 presents how to apply the four vital stages in dealing with the disturbance of Mr Khanna.

Box 4.1

Sample of Implementation of Four Vital Stages of REBT

First stage: Identification of correct self-talk

1. How can he say that he is short of cash?
2. It is his duty to reimburse my taxi fare; therefore, he *must* not have refused to settle my bill.
3. At least in the future, the clerk *must* not refuse to settle my bill.
4. It is awful that he is not ready to do what he is supposed to do.
5. I cannot tolerate this situation.
6. He is silly fool and therefore, he *must* be condemned and punished. Being a silly fool, he will always harass me in the future too.

Second stage: Identification of core irrational belief

As I very much want all human beings to treat me kindly and justly, they invariably *should* and *must* behave accordingly. Or else, they are useless people, who deserve to be completely condemned and punished.

(Box 4.1 Continued)

(Box 4.1 Continued)

Third stage: Disputation (Example)

Is it not absurd to say that he *must* not have refused to settle my bill because as a matter of fact, he did refuse to settle my bill. Does it not fly in the face of reality to say that he *must* not have done what he actually did?

Fourth stage: Replacement of rational belief

Human beings are free to behave as they wish to. No law of the universe compels them to behave in any specific way.

REBT Today

Since Ellis presented the original version of his system of psychotherapy in 1955, it has undergone some revisions periodically.

Changes in the title (RT, RET and REBT): As Windy Dryden said, rational when used in RT, means 'that which helps people to achieve their basic goals and purposes whereas "irrational" means that which prevents them from achieving these goals and purposes' (Ellis & Maclaren, 2003). In short, rational means self-helping and irrational means self-defeating.

Many critics were not ready to accept the meanings of the words 'rational' and 'irrational' in their simplified forms described by Dryden. The reason is that the word 'rational' is perceived differently by different people. General misconception is that rational means unemotional. Ellis was criticized consistently for neglecting emotive aspect of psychological disturbance.

Nevertheless, in view of this persistent charge, in 1961, Ellis changed the title of his system from 'RT' to 'RET'. Finally, in 1993, he again changed even this new name to 'REBT' in order to make it clear that his system of psychotherapy does not neglect the behavioural component of psychological disturbance. In keeping with this changed name, the institute's name was also changed to 'Albert Ellis Institute for Rational Emotive Therapy' and finally even this name was changed to 'Albert Ellis Institute'.

It does not mean that Ellis changed the name of his system of psychotherapy to appease his critics. As said earlier, from the very beginning, he had been reiterating that cognitive, emotive and behavioural processes are not separate. For instance, when a student has a very low opinion of his abilities, he is likely to feel inadequate and act differently. Conversely, if he feels inadequate, he is likely to entertain negative thoughts about himself and act diffidently. When he acts diffidently, he is likely to create a low opinion about himself and feel inadequate. This proves Ellis' view that cognition, emotion and behaviour are not independent psychological processes but rather are highly interdependent and interactive processes.

Incidentally, the current name of Ellis's system of psychotherapy, namely, 'Rational Emotive Behaviour Therapy' was not the instantaneous discovery. In 1974, in his foreword to Dr Donald Tosi's book, *Youth: Toward Personal Growth: A Rational-Emotive Approach* (Tosi, 1974), Ellis had mentioned that RET could be easily called something such as REBT or Rational Behaviour Therapy (RBT) as some of its adherents prefer to call it. This clearly exhibits that many years before he actually changed the title, he was ruminating over it.

Suffice it to say that Ellis changed the name of his therapeutic system two times for making the theoretical underpinnings of his treatment strategy more explicit, not just to pacify his critics.

Humanistic philosophy: REBT is just not a scientific system that helps people get rid of their emotional disturbance and live a more productive and happy life. If this were the only goal of REBT, it would have two major components:

1. Causes of emotional disturbance
2. A bunch of therapeutic techniques

REBT is something more than a scientific and technique-bound system of psychotherapy. From the very beginning, it has emphasized how a man's faulty, that is, irrational philosophy of life makes him emotionally disturbed and how his improvement will not only require a behavioural change in him but also a profound philosophical change. Therefore, it does not restrict itself to the causes and cures of emotional disturbance. It helps develop not just a rational but a humane philosophy of life too. In fact, this philosophical component of REBT is its third and most distinguishing component. This third component of REBT can be called

3. A humanistic philosophy of life

In view of this consideration, REBT is described today under three major headings and not just two headings corresponding to the aforementioned two components. During the last 60 years or so, the growth of REBT has been phenomenal. Its insightful journey during the past six decades will be unfolded as we proceed further.

References

Ellis, A. (1968). What really causes therapeutic change? *Voices, 4*(2), 90–97.

———. (1974). Rational-emotive therapy. In A. Burton (Ed.), *Operational Theories of Personality.* New York, NY: Brunner/Mazel.

———. (1979). The theory of rational-emotive therapy. In A. Ellis & J. Whiteley (Eds.), *Theoretical and Empirical Foundations of Rational-Emotive Therapy* (p. 45). California, CA: Brooks/Cole Publishing Company.

———. (1994). *Reason and Emotion in Psychotherapy: A Comprehensive Method of Treating Human Disturbances Revised and Updated.* New York, NY: Carol Publishing.

Ellis, A., & Grieger, R. (1977). *Handbook of Rational-Emotive Therapy.* New York, NY: Springer.

Ellis, A., & Maclaren, C. (2003). *Rational Emotive Behavior Therapy: A Therapist's Guide* (p. 19). Fourth Reprint. California, CA: Impact Publishers.

Phadke, K.M. & Khear, R. (2001). *The Inner World of Entrepreneurs: Improving Relationship of Work and at Home* (p. 27). Mumbai: Pauline Publications.

Tosi, D. (1974). *Youth: Toward Personal Growth: A Rational Emotive Approach.* Counselling Youth Series. New York: Merrill Publishers.

Walen, S.R., DiGiuseppe, R., & Wessler, R.L. (1980). *A Practitioner's Guide to Rational-Emotive Therapy* (pp. 13–15). New York, NY: Oxford University Press.

Further Readings

Dryden, W. (Ed.). (1990). *The Essential Albert Ellis.* New York: Springer.

Ellis, A. (1996). *Better, Deeper, and More Enduring Brief Therapy.* New York, NY: Brunner/Mazel.

McGinn, L.K., & Ellis, A. (1997). Interview: Albert Ellis on Rational Emotive Behavior Therapy. *American Journal of Psychotherapy, 51*(3), 309–16.

Phadke, K.M. (1999). *Adhunik Sanjivani.* Mumbai: Tridal Prakashan.

5

Critical Analysis of Psychological Disturbance

In this chapter, we will discuss the meaning and causes of psychological disturbance. For this, we will study three hypothetical cases, namely, Aditi, Vikram and Saniya. All three of them are emotionally upset. We will see how REBT looks at their emotional disturbance. While analysing their disturbance from the REBT point of view, we will use words such as emotional disturbance, psychological disturbance and mental disturbance synonymously.

In Chapter 4, we already got acquainted with 'ABC'. In this chapter, we will see the expansion of 'A'. Some light will be thrown on 'B' and further details of 'B' and 'C' will be reviewed in Chapter 6.

Three Cases of Emotional Disturbance

Case 5.1

Case of Aditi

Aditi, a 20-year-old graduate in computer science, has been trying to get a suitable job for quite some time. In reply to her application for a job, a multinational company has called her for an interview. However, she is anxious about going for the interview and facing a panel of experts in computer science. Of course, she knows very well that if she wants a job, she has to go for the interview. Yet, she is feeling anxious and wants to avoid going for the interview. Her main psychological disturbance is anxiety.

Case 5.2

Case of Vikram

Vikram is a 27-years-old accountant. He is good at his work and has excellent career prospects in his company. However, he is fed up with his boss, who, according to him, uses dictatorial methods to get him to do work. Therefore, he is so angry at his boss that he does not feel like going to work every morning. At the same time, he is aware that as per his contract with the company, he cannot leave his job until the next year. Also, he knows that because of his present financial and family conditions, it would be self-defeating to leave his job at the moment. Vikram's main psychological disturbance is anger.

Case 5.3

Case of Saniya

Twenty-five-year-old Saniya is of medium height. Moreover, her weight is much more than the normal weight for her age and height. Hence, her doctor has advised her to reduce her weight by at least 5 kg. The doctor has also prescribed her a special diet which will help her reduce her weight. She has learned through experience that by following the doctor's advice, even for about a month, she will be able to reduce her weight considerably. Yet, she is unable to follow the doctor's advice regularly over a long time. After that, she gives up dieting and begins to eat and drink to her heart's content. As a result, she feels depressed and inert; or, she becomes rebellious and gives up her goal of reducing her weight by 5 kg. Saniya's main psychological disturbance is depression.

The three cases (Cases 5.1–5.3) are very common and we often meet many people in our daily life who resemble them to a large extent. In a way, these cases are representative cases of our society. Hence, they will be referred in subsequent chapters too in order to explain various other components of REBT.

Man's Struggle for Goal-seeking

A basic premise of REBT is that human beings are disturbed when their goal-seeking activities are thwarted. If they always achieve their goals, they will obviously have no reason to feel disturbed.

Let us therefore begin with the letter G, which in REBT stands for the main goals or purposes people pursue. Of course, broadly speaking, they are two: (a) people struggle to stay alive and (b) people want to remain happy. These two obvious goals include several other goals. For example, people want to enjoy life, sometimes by themselves and sometimes by seeking the company of others. Usually they also choose to have intimate relations with at least a few other people. Besides, they often try to find some meaning in life. As a result, they pursue some vocational, religious, spiritual and humanitarian objectives. They may select and follow some recreational goals too. This is, by no means, an exhaustive list of goals human beings seek to achieve. However, even to pursue these goals, they have to set several short-term and long-term goals. Yet it goes without saying that they seek happiness and avoid unhappiness. When they encounter obstacles in their path, they tend to become emotionally disturbed. REBT can be understood easily if we try to conceptualize the disturbances of Aditi, Vikram and Saniya in terms of therapeutic framework.

Analysis of Cases 5.1, 5.2 and 5.3 in Terms of Therapeutic Framework

Aditi: Aditi's goal (G) is to get a suitable job. However, the situation that thwarts her goal-seeking behaviour is that she is called for an interview. It is called an 'activating' event, activating experience or adversity (denoted by the letter A). Her psychological disturbance, namely, the anxiety in her mind, is called a consequence (denoted by the letter C). Her 'view' of this event in her life is called her belief (denoted by the letter B). What is her belief (B) about the prospect of facing the interviewers? She interprets the interview as an event that will expose her ignorance. According to her evaluative criterion, her ignorance will prove that she is a worthless human being and that would be terrible and unbearable.

Vikram: Vikram's goal (G) is to pursue a good career path available to him in his company or to stay in the current job for at least a year. Let us understand his emotional disturbance by following the ABC theory. The methods Vikram's boss adopts to get the work done from him are called Activating events, or Activating experiences, or Adversities (denoted by the letter A). Vikram's anger at his boss is called a Consequence (denoted by the letter C). Vikram's view of his boss' methods of getting work done from him is called his Belief (denoted by the letter B). What is Vikram's belief (B) about his boss' methods of getting work done from him? He interprets those methods as dictatorial and therefore unfair. According to his evaluative criterion, his boss is useless because he uses dictatorial and unfair methods for getting work done from him.

Saniya: Saniya's goal (G) is to follow her doctor's advice in order to reduce her weight by 5 kg. The diet that her doctor has prescribed to her is an Activating event, or Activating experience or Adversity (denoted by the letter A). Her view of the prescribed diet is called her Belief (denoted by the letter B). What is her belief (B) about the diet prescribed by her doctor? She interprets the prescribed diet as too difficult to follow regularly for a long time. According to her evaluative criterion, it is pitiable that she is expected to follow such an unfair advice of her doctor.

Even these cursory conceptualization of the emotional disturbance of all three in terms of REBT framework is enough to highlight a very important message of REBT: Our emotional disturbance (C) is not directly caused by the adversities in our life (A); rather, it is largely caused by the way we view those adversities (B).

Analysis of Psychological Disturbance

ABC framework can be easily understood with help of Box 5.1.

Box 5.1

Arithmetical Expression of ABC Framework

Common Perception

Emotional disturbance is created by outside events or people.

A--C

ABC framework in REBT

Emotional disturbance is largely created by irrational beliefs towards outside events or people.

$$A \times B = C$$

This arithmetical expression of ABC shows that emotional disturbance (C) is the product of multiplication of activating event (A) by irrational belief (B).

In Box 5.1, the common perception of the cause of disturbance is shown by letters 'A' and 'C'. In the REBT model, the addition of the letter 'B' signifies the importance of beliefs in emotional disturbance.

Multiplication sign: Why is the relation between A and C shown by a multiplication sign in the ABC framework of REBT? Why is the sign of 'addition' insufficient to indicate the relation? In order to get these answers, let us discuss the significance of these signs further. Suppose we add 3 and 6, the answer will be 9. Instead of adding, if we multiply 3 by 6 the answer is 18, which suggests that there is a multiple increase in the quantity of the product. Ellis used the same analogy when he used multiplication sign while analysing ABC. What he meant is when something happens at 'A', we simply do not add the beliefs into the events but multiply them instead. The product we get at 'C' is much larger and disproportionate to 'A'. We end up paying the huge cost of emotional consequences unnecessarily. Box 5.2 will explain this more clearly.

Box 5.2

Revised Arithmetical Expression of ABC Framework

$$A \times B = C$$

This revised expression shows that when we multiply Activating Event (A) by Irrational Belief (B), the product we get of Emotional Disturbance (C) is incommensurable.

Box 5.2 presents the increased magnitude of 'C'. Many a times, the event that occurs at 'A' is trivial but at point 'C', we experience severe emotional disturbance that is not proportional to the magnitude of 'A'. This stresses the significance of multiplication.

Of course, we need to remember that this arithmetical expression is used just to show how the enormity of 'C' is self-created. The objective is not to discuss the arithmetic models of multiplication or what if the operator is decimal number. The only objective here is to show how the multiplication creates a bigger impact.

Role of Activating Event

Analysis of Cases 5.1, 5.2 and 5.3: The ABC theory does not state or imply that a man's emotional disturbance (C) has nothing to do with the adversities (A) in his life. What the theory asserts is that by itself, A does not cause C. For example, unlike Aditi, some people, when called for an interview, do not experience anxiety. Some people feel happy when they are called for an interview. Similarly, some people whose boss' methods are just like that of Vikram's boss don't seethe with anger. Some learn to cope with the boss' methods, whereas some may even adopt those very methods while getting the work done from their own subordinates. Finally, if many girls are prescribed exactly the same diet that Saniya's doctor prescribed to her, not all of them might feel depressed like Saniya. Some of them may even feel enthusiastic about following the prescribed diet.

In view of these variations in the emotional responses of people to the same circumstances, the ABC theory proposes that the belief of a man, coupled with the surrounding circumstances give rise to his emotional responses. In other words, the adversities in a man's life help him choose his emotions. They do not make him choose what he chooses. He is responsible for choosing his emotions at least to some extent.

Suppose Aditi does not want a job. She will not apply for a job in any company and therefore will not receive a call for an interview. But a call for the interview makes her feel anxious because she already holds a belief about facing interviewers. If Vikram is not bothered about pursuing a good career path available in his company or if he does not have the necessity of staying in his company for at least a year, then his boss' methods of getting the work done from him will not make him seethe with anger. The methods his boss adopts for getting work done from him make him fume with anger because he already holds a belief about fair and unfair methods of getting the work done from subordinates. If Saniya is not interested in following the advice of her doctor in order to reduce her weight by 5 kg, she will not feel depressed because she already holds a belief regarding the kind of diet she can follow regularly for a long time.

The account of Ellis' ABC theory of emotional disturbance given here is admittedly sketchy. The subsequent parts of this book will put flesh on the bare bones of A, B and C presented here. Even this rough outline of Ellis' ABC theory is enough to suggest that human beings have some choice over their emotional responses to the adversities in life. They are not completely helpless in the face of adversities. Another way of putting this message is that when humans are confronted with trying circumstances, they can, at least to a certain degree, choose their emotions. Therefore, with the help of ABC theory, they can choose to empower themselves.

More About Activating Events

The broad outline of the ABC theory previously presented in this book is enough to demonstrate the pivotal role Ellis ascribes to a man's point of view or philosophy of life in the creation and maintenance of his emotional disturbance. However, the apparent simplicity of the theory is somewhat deceptive. The letters A, B and C in the ABC theory are symbols that represent complex factors. Therefore, it is necessary to go into the details of those complexities systematically so as to understand the full significance of Ellis' view of man's emotional disturbance.

Let us begin with the first letter, that is, A, in the ABC theory. Of course, the letter A stands for activating event, activating experience or adversity in the ABC theory. There are different types of activating events, however. For example, a declining physical condition, a possibility of bankruptcy, a threat of imprisonment, etc. can serve as activating events for some people. Similarly, for some people, activating events are the behaviours of their family members, neighbours, shopkeepers, government officers, in-laws, etc., whereas scheduled dates for completing assignments, studying to get a university degree, regularly maintaining records of their income and expenditure, etc. can be activating events for some others. All these kinds of people will create different emotions in their minds according to their beliefs about the activating events in their lives.

Indeed, activating events are countless. Human beings experience different emotions when they encounter any one of the countless activating events because they hold different beliefs about that particular activating event.

One more clarification about activating events is necessary. Activating events can be good, indifferent or bad. However, people rarely seek psychological help when they meet good activating events in their lives. Usually, they seek psychological help to cope with bad or adverse activating events in their lives. That is why activating events or activating experiences are called adversities.

Multiple Features of Activating Events

Activating events have a number of features. We will examine these features in the context of Cases 5.1, 5.2 and 5.3.

Actual or Imagined 'A'

'A' can be an actual event: If activating events happen in reality and can be observed, they are considered as actual events. For example, In Aditi's case, reading a call letter for an interview from a company; in Vikram's case, his boss' order to him to do a particular work and the diet prescribed by Saniya's doctor are actual activating events. These events are observable and can be tested out.

'A' can be imagined: If actual activating events trigger other inferences or interpretations about the events in our lives, then they can be considered as 'imagined activating events'. These inferences go beyond observable data which may be correct or incorrect, but they are personally significant to the person and therefore lead to emotional disturbance. For example, When Aditi reads a call letter for an interview, she starts imagining that she is unable to answer the questions asked by interview panellist and gets anxious. Here, activating event is imagined. In Vikram's case, what he infers from his boss' order is that he is disrespecting him and gets angry. In this case too, the activating event is imagined. Similarly, in Saniya's case, by seeing the prescription of the diet given by her doctor if she imagines that she will be unable to follow it, she feels depressed. This is another case where the activating event is imagined.

Present, Past and Future 'A'

Activating events are further classified as present, past and future activating events.

Present 'A': If the person is experiencing the activating event currently, it is classified as 'present activating event'. For example, an activating event in Aditi's life is reading a call letter for the interview. This event has occurred in her life right now. In Vikram's life, the activating event at the moment is his boss' order to get work done. What is an activating event in Saniya's life at the present time? It is the diet prescribed by her doctor. All the activating events in these cases are present ones.

Past 'A': Aditi, Vikram and Saniya can be stimulated if they recall the activating events which took place in the past. For instance, Aditi can recall how she had fumbled in oral examinations during her academic career. The memories of those events form her past can become activating events in her life now. Depending on her current beliefs about fumbling in oral examinations, she will create some emotions in her mind. Similarly, Vikram can brood on the methods his boss had used to get the work done from him about a year ago. As a result of this, brooding over those past events can become activating events in his life right now. According to his current beliefs about methods of getting work done from his subordinates, he will experience some emotions now. Saniya can recall her experience of unsuccessful efforts to follow the diet prescribed by her doctor. This memory of her experience can become an activating event in her life right now. As per her current belief about dieting, she will create some emotions in her mind. All activating events in these cases are past ones.

Future 'A': There is yet another type of activating events. It consists of events that may occur in the future. Human beings imagine the events that can take place in the years to come. For instance, Aditi can imagine what would happen if she always avoids to go to job interviews. Depending on her belief about such a possibility, she will experience some emotions now. Similarly, Vikram can imagine what his career would be like if he is destined to work all his life under bosses whose methods are unfair. Depending on his belief about such a possibility, he will experience some emotions. Saniya too can imagine what would happen to her health if she never implements any prescribed diet regularly for a long time. Depending on her belief about such a possibility, she will create some emotions in her mind.

Critical or Inferential 'A'

Windy Dryden (2013) presented REBT's situational ABC model in which he proposed that a situation is the description of an actual event or fact. A critical event is the inference that people derive from actual events, which evoke their emotional responses. Hence, Critical A is that aspect of the situation when people experience emotional responses. This model makes the distinction between Critical A (which evokes emotional response) and the situation (actual event). Critical A includes inferential meaning whereas situations do not include this meaning.

In Aditi's case, reading a call letter for an interview, is the situation (description of the fact or event) while Critical A is the interview which is hard to crack (inferences the person has made about the situation). In Vikram's case, his boss' order is the situation while the understanding that his words are offensive is critical A. In Saniya's example, the diet prescribed by her doctor is the situation while the diet being too stringent to follow is Critical A.

The model further describes that these inferences can be true or false. In order to decide the truth, a person has to evaluate his inferences against available evidence. Aditi, Vikram and Saniya will also evaluate their interferences against the evidence such as their experiences, other's experiences, their own performances and so on.

More about Beliefs

The letter B in the ABC theory of emotional disturbance denotes a man's beliefs. In response to a given activating event, people produce different emotions in their minds largely because they hold different beliefs about that activating event. According to the ABC theory, a man's beliefs include many factors. For example, they include, or amount to include, his explicit or implicit point of view or his philosophy of life. That is why Ellis often interpreted the letter B in the ABC theory as Belief System. Surely, the phrase Belief System more aptly describes the role that a man's philosophy of life plays in the creation and continuation of his emotional disturbance.

Acquisition of Beliefs

When it is said that a man has a belief in XYZ, it means that he has an idea that XYZ is true. How does he come to accept the idea that XYZ is true? How does he acquire that idea? Ellis has mentioned three sources by which we acquire these ideas or beliefs.

1. **Family and society:** It is the most primary source of acquisition of beliefs. In the process of growing up in the family, a man starts acquiring the beliefs that are prevalent in the members of his family. Many beliefs are suggested to him by his parents, teachers and other forces in the society. When he accepts those prevalent beliefs, he finds it easy to adjust to the members of his family and the social world around him and thereby reach his goals, whereas if he goes against the beliefs held by the significant people in his environment, he meets with obstacles and even penalties which make it difficult for him to reach his goals.

   There is another aspect to the process of acquiring beliefs. As man is not capable of thinking for himself in his childhood, he accepts whatever is taught to him by the members of his family and the other significant people in his socio-cultural environment. That is why La Barre (1955, p. 106), a well-known sociologist, has cryptically remarked, 'A child per force becomes a Right Thinker, before he begins to think at all'.

Ellis agrees with the idea that the origin of man's beliefs can be traced back to the socio-cultural world in which he is born and brought up. He also points out two additional factors that influence and shape a man's beliefs.

2. **Biological disposition:** All children born in a given society do not completely accept all the beliefs prevalent in their socio-cultural environment. This is because every child is born with his unique innate tendency to be suggestible or teachable and to easily pick up the customs and traditions of that given society. Some children easily accept most of the ideas of others compared to other children in the same society. Hence, children differ in their biological predisposition to be suggestible or teachable.

3. **Self-creation:** A man is born with the ability to think about and review the beliefs taught to him. He does not always blindly swallow whatever is taught to him. He is also born with the ability to think creatively. He often manufactures or invents his own beliefs. Thus, even from his childhood, he has some choice about accepting or rejecting the ideas drummed into him continually. In fact, psychotherapy endeavours to bring about a change in people's self-defeating, and other-defeating thinking, because it presumes that people have some choice about what to think and how to think.

Manifestation of Beliefs

Many thoughts are constantly running in our mind. There is an ongoing dialogue in our mind all day long. For example, while reading this text also, some thoughts *must* have passed your mind. You *must* have thought about the meaning of the text, whether to agree with the meaning or different interpretations of this text among other things. If we turn our awareness inward, we will realize that whenever we think, we actually have a conversation with ourselves. It is called self-talk. Self-talk is a psychological term for all the things that a person tells himself.

Self-talk: Our beliefs are manifested by our self-talk. In self-talk we use words, phrases and sentences to communicate with ourselves and thereby our core beliefs and philosophies of life and also our secondary derivatives. In other words, what we talk to ourselves, that is, our self-sentences provide a good clue to what irrational beliefs or philosophies we not only hold but also go on drumming into our mind. Emotions result largely from what we tell ourselves.

Obstruction in problem solving in reference to Case 5.3: Self-talk creates some unnecessary and troublesome emotional difficulties in connection with their objective problems. Let us review Saniya's case to get a clarification on this point. The moment her doctor advises her to reduce weight, she begins to tell herself the following sentences regarding the practical problem of reducing her weight by 5 kg: 'How easy it is for the doctor to advise me to reduce my weight! But is it really so easy to reduce my weight by 5 kg? Who says that thin people have good health? Will I really benefit by shedding my weight?' Thus, Saniya creates an emotion of senseless rebellion in her mind.

Then she further says to herself: 'I have been eating rich food from childhood. I cannot live without it ... Now it is impossible for me to stop eating it'. So, in way, she creates the emotion of inadequacy and diffidence in her mind.

This is what she tells herself subsequently: 'Let me suppose that for reducing my weight, I make strenuous efforts to follow the diet prescribed by the doctor. If after some days, I fail to implement the entire regimen meticulously...' This is how she creates the emotion of anxiety in her mind.

After some days, she talks to herself in this way: 'From the first of this month I tried to control my habit of eating. But today on the fourth day, I ate too much oily food ... and took two ice creams too. Oh! I have failed to restrain my mind! I am a good for nothing person. I have not even been able to do such an easy thing like dieting ... What a stupid girl I am!' These sentences generate emotions of worthlessness, depression and inferiority in her mind.

Her self-talk then continues in this manner: 'But what is the necessity of reducing my weight? Even if I reduce my weight, how long am I going to live after all ... Can the doctor give me any guarantee that all my problems about my health will be over?' This leads to the feeling of inertia and she once again proclaims her senseless rebellion.

Have you noticed how Saniya creates harmful and unnecessary emotional problems in her mind because of what she talks to herself? As a result of everything she talks to herself, her practical problem of reducing weight gets literally engulfed in the whirlwind of her emotions. Her main practical problem and her self-created needless emotional problems about the main problem will be clearly understood from Figure 5.1.

Figure 5.1

Obstruction in Problem Solving

Senseless Rebellion		
Inferiority	Practical Problem: How do I reduce my weight by 5 kg?	Anxiety
	Self-Talk ↓ Obstruction in practical problem solving	Self-hatred
Depression and worthlessness		

Figure 5.1 presents how Saniya's practical problem is engulfed in the whirlwind of self-defeating emotions such as inferiority, anxiety, self-hatred, depression and worthlessness.

Characteristics of Self-talk: Identification of correct self-talk is very important tool in REBT to detect irrational beliefs. However, this identification is very challenging. It is not always an accurate index of the meanings we give to the adversities in our life. Moreover, we are not aware about our accurate self-talk. The reason lies in some peculiar characteristics of self-talk.

1. *Speed:* Self-talk occurs at a very high speed, making it difficult to bring into awareness. We talk to ourselves almost 600–800 words per minute. Hence, it is difficult for people to remember all the words and content of their self-talk.
2. *Preconscious state:* Most of our self-talk occurs at a preconscious level. In other words, we are not fully aware about our precise self-talk. However, it does not mean that we will never be aware about the sentences we utter to ourselves. With the consistent efforts and usage of tools and techniques, we can bring it to the conscious level.
3. *Abbreviated form:* Many of the self-sentences appear in abbreviated form. When something happens at 'A', we do not utter all the sentences related to the implied meaning. We utter only few key words, but they carry all implied meanings. For example, if the car

passes us just by two inches, we utter to ourselves, 'Oh, My God!' These three words actually contain thousands of sentences. The abbreviated form of self-talk makes the process of its identification tough.

Images: When REBT was a very young discipline in the late 1950s, Ellis emphasized that a man's irrational self-talk made him emotionally disturbed. Ellis gradually modified his views and began to make it clear that man's emotional disturbance was largely (not completely) created by the faulty meanings and philosophies he kept on communicating to himself when confronted with the adversities in his life. These meanings can be traced through self-talk and images. This shift in Ellis's emphasis was a result of his observation that the meanings a disturbed man gave to the adversities in his life and the philosophies underlying those meanings were not always manifested in the words, phrases and sentences he went on telling himself.

Ellis concluded that along with sentences, man's meaning frequently takes the form of images, symbols and other forms of communicating with himself. In short, the beliefs are manifested by images too. Nevertheless, the person can be made aware of those meanings and the philosophies underlying them with some patience and efforts. Hence, in the present version of REBT, more importance is given to the meanings a disturbed man gives to the adversities in his life and the philosophies which bolster them up through self-talk and images.

Rational and Irrational Beliefs

If the ABC theory states that a man's emotional disturbance is largely caused by his beliefs, his belief system or his philosophy of life, it becomes imperative to ask which beliefs or philosophies of life lie at the root of human emotional disturbance. Surely, sensible or rational beliefs or philosophies of life cannot be expected to give rise to disturbing emotions such as anger, hostility, anxiety, guilt, depression, etc. It goes without saying that a man's emotional disturbance is caused by his senseless or irrational beliefs or philosophies of life.

REBT aims at helping the disturbed people overcome their irrational beliefs and begin to live a healthier life by inculcating rational beliefs. Hence, it is mainly interested in understanding two types of beliefs— senseless or irrational beliefs and sensible or rational beliefs. However, it does not mean that all beliefs can be divided into these two categories. Those other beliefs are not very relevant in understanding and overcoming psychological disturbance.

Therefore, REBT focuses on a man's irrational beliefs in order to diagnose and cure his emotional disturbance. This implies that REBT can give a precise definition of rationality. As Ellis himself admits, it is not possible to give any absolute definition of rationality, although a workable definition of rationality can be given. For example, thinking which helps people in reaching their goals can be considered rational, whereas thinking which blocks the attainment of their goals can be called irrational. In short, self-helping thinking is rational and self-defeating thinking is irrational.

Criteria for Rational Thinking

In 1975 Dr Maxie C. Maultsby, Jr (1986), a psychiatrist, presented a more refined version of what could be considered rational thinking. In fact, he gave the rules of rational thinking: People who think irrationally

1. often perceive things wrongly.
2. endanger their own safety.
3. hinder their progress towards their own goals again and again.
4. create mental agitation which makes them feel quite uncomfortable.
5. create unnecessary conflicts between themselves and other people.

In 1968, he had visited the Albert Ellis Institute to study REBT with Ellis and had spent a lot of time there with a view to studying Ellis' style of working with individuals and groups. After returning to Madison, Wisconsin, he developed and continued to practise his own modified version of REBT called RBT.

The five rules or criteria of rational thinking propounded by Dr Maxie C. Maultsby, Jr, were accepted by Ellis and also incorporated in the third edition of the book, *A Guide to Rational Living* (Ellis & Harper, 1997). Following are the five criteria of rational thinking:

1. Rational thinking is based on the facts or reality.
2. Rational thinking protects our health and life.
3. Rational thinking takes us towards a goal.
4. Rational thinking eliminates our unwanted mental conflict.
5. Rational thinking eliminates unwanted conflict with others.

These criteria are useful to determine if a thought or behaviour is rational or irrational. In the context of these questions, Ellis came up with the clarification on what he meant by rational thinking and its implications in REBT (Tosi, 1979). Rational thinking has to do with logically correct thinking that considers facts and their interrelationships according to commonly accepted rules. It portrays rational thinking as a way of achieving some long-term constructive goal or a set of goals. It also helps the person minimize his mental conflict and get better. When applied to beliefs, the term 'rational' has following five defining characteristics (Dryden & Branch, 2008):

1. Flexible or non-extreme
2. Consistent with reality
3. Logical
4. Largely functional in their emotional, behavioural and cognitive consequences
5. Largely helpful to the individual in pursuing his basic goals and purposes

Simplified version: Ellis later reviewed these characteristics and simplified the criteria of rational thinking by reducing them to three. According to him, a practitioner of REBT can assess whether his client's thinking is rational or irrational by examining it in the light of questions (Ellis, 1999) presented in Table 5.1.

The present version of REBT contains following checkpoints for rationality:

1. *Functional or pragmatic*—rational beliefs help the person in the long run to reach his goal and feel better.

Table 5.1

Three Criteria for Rationality and Irrationality

No.	Criterion
1.	Does it help the client over the long run to believe this? If it hinders, what thought would help him reach his goals better and feel better?
2.	Is the client's thinking consistent with the facts? If it isn't, what is?
3.	Is the client's thinking logical? If not, what would make more sense logically?

'Yes' answers to the first part of all three questions indicate the thought is rational. If the answer is 'no', then we need to deal with the second part.

Source: Ellis et al. (2003).

2. *Factual or empirical*—rational beliefs are consistent with the facts.
3. *Logical or non-absolutist*—rational beliefs are logical.

Conversely, three criteria for irrationality are as follows:

1. *Non-functional or non-pragmatic*—irrational beliefs prevent people from achieving their basic goals and purposes.
2. *Non-factual or non-empirical*—irrational beliefs are empirically inconsistent with reality.
3. *Illogical or absolutist*—irrational beliefs are illogical, dogmatic and masturbatory.

This checklist provides a handy tool for identifying objectively rational and irrational beliefs and behaviour. However, if the person follows even the first two criteria, his thinking is considered rational.

Many people have a difficulty in checking the first criterion of factual thinking. The problem is that what they sincerely believe to be true is not necessarily factual. They dogmatically convince themselves of their truth and ignore evidence that contradicts their hypotheses. One technique to help determine whether the thinking is based on fact is the Camera Check of Perceptions (Pucci, 2006). In this technique, one has to ask himself, 'If I were to take a picture of the situation, I am describing to myself, or if I were to use a video camera to record it and played the tape back, would it show what I am saying about the situation?' This technique does not only help us confirm that we have our facts straight but also helps us confirm that we say what we mean and mean what we say to ourselves.

In short, REBT helps the person discriminate between rational and irrational beliefs. It holds that rational beliefs normally lead to healthy and irrational beliefs to unhealthy emoting. Rational beliefs, and healthy feelings and behaviours, are socially interested and help preserve, perpetuate and enhance the happiness of the group in which the person chooses to live and of the human race as a whole (Ellis & Harper, 1975).

References

Dryden, W. (2013). *Rationality & Pluralism: The Selected Works of Windy Dryden* (pp. 153–54). (World Library of Mental Health). New York, NY: Routledge.

Dryden, W., & Branch, R. (2008). *The Fundamentals of Rational Emotive Behaviour Therapy: A Training Handbook* (2nd edition, p. 8). West Sussex: John Wiley & Sons.

Ellis, A. (1999). *Make Yourself Happy and Remarkably Less Disturbable.* Mumbai: Jaico Publishing House.

Ellis, A., Gordon J., Neenan, M., & Palmer S. (2003). *Stress Counseling: A Rational Emotive Behaviour Approach* (p. 5). Continuum, New York, NY: SAGE.

Ellis, A., & Harper, R. (1975). *A Guide to Rational Living* (p. 28). California, CA: Melvin Powers Wilshire.

————. (1997). *A Guide to Rational Living* (3rd edition). California, CA: Melvin Powers Wilshire.

La Barre, W. (1955). The human animal. In A. Ellis (Ed.), *Reason and Emotion in Psychotherapy: A Comprehensive Method of Treating Human Disturbances* (p. 106). (Revised and updated). New York: Carol Publishing.

Maultsby, Maxie C., Jr. (1986). *Coping Better... Anytime, Anywhere: The Handbook of Rational Self-Counseling.* Alexandria, Virginia: RBT Center, LTC.

Pucci, A. (2006). *The Client's Guide to Cognitive-Behavioral Therapy: How to Live a Healthy Happy Life, No Matter What* (pp. 42–43). New York: Universe.

Tosi, D. (1979). Personality reactions with some emphasis on new directions application and research. In A. Ellis, J.M. Whiteley (Eds.), *Theoretical and Empirical Foundations of Rational-Emotive Therapy* (p. 182). Brooks/Cole Series in Counseling Psychology. Monterey, CA: Brooks/Cole.

Further Readings

Ellis, A. (1972). Helping people get better than merely feel better. *Rational Living, 7*(2), 2–9.

————. (1991). Using RET effectively: Reflections and interview. In M.E. Bernard (Ed.), *Using Rational-Emotive Therapy Effectively* (pp. 1–33). New York, NY: Plenum.

Phadke, K.M. (1999). *Adhunik Sanjivani.* Mumbai: Tridal Prakashan.

6

Irrational Beliefs: Nature and Review

In the previous chapters, we have seen how psychological disturbance is largely created by irrational beliefs. Now we will turn our attention to the analysis of major irrational beliefs. We will also see the letter 'C' from ABC framework in more detail.

Hallmark of Irrationality

When Ellis began to use his self-created system of psychotherapy, namely, rational therapy, in 1955, he surely did not have a readymade list of the irrational beliefs which make people emotionally disturbed. Rather, as a result of his clinical experiences, he gradually began to systematically formulate the irrational beliefs which his clients expressed through their disturbing emotions such as anxiety, guilt, self-pity, anger, hostility, depression, rebellion and what not. Then, as we have seen earlier, in his paper on rational therapy which he presented at the Annual Convention of the APA in Chicago on 31 August 1956, he gave a list of 12 irrational beliefs and their rational counterparts.

However, as he gained more and more clinical experience, he came to the conclusion that there was one common factor in all the irrational beliefs to which his clients subscribed. That common factor was the rigid demandingness implicit in all irrational beliefs. This demandingness is expressed in the form of *musts*, absolute *shoulds*, have to's, got to's, etc. Ellis concluded that our dogmatic *musts* or demands are at the core of psychological disturbance. To clarify this point, let us consider our three cases again.

Analysis of Cases 5.1, 5.2 and 5.3: Aditi is anxious because she implicitly believes that her ignorance *must not* or *should not* be exposed while facing the interviewers. Vikram's tacit belief is that his boss *must not* or *should not* use dictatorial methods of getting work done from him. He is hence angry with his boss. Saniya is feeling depressed because, in her heart, she seems to nurture the belief that the diet prescribed by her doctor *must not* or *should not* be difficult to follow for a long time.

Eventually, Ellis could easily see the explicit or implicit *must, should* or ought underlying his client's emotional disturbance. Thus, he arrived at the conclusion that when clients make rigid demands as to how they themselves *must* behave, how others *must* behave and how the conditions surrounding them *must* be, they become emotionally upset.

In fact, Ellis developed the idea that when people turn their desires, wants, wishes and preferences to rigid, inflexible and absolutistic demands, commands, *shoulds*, oughts and *musts*, they become emotionally disturbed. Ellis humorously termed this way of thinking by a word that he coined himself—*musturbation*. The word *musturbation* refers to people believing that something *must or must not* happen.

As Ellis felt more and more convinced that human beings become emotionally disturbed when they believe that something *must* or *must* not happen, he carefully reviewed his original list of 12 irrational beliefs. Then, he came to the conclusion that those 12 irrational beliefs could be rephrased and also reclassified more logically. A man can indulge in *musturbation* in three ways. First, he can believe what he himself *must* do and *must not* do. Second, he can believe what others *must* do and *must not* do. Third, he can believe how the conditions around him *must* be and *must not* be. Therefore, from 1977, Ellis began to present irrational beliefs or irrational philosophies of life under the three musturbatory ideologies.

Three Musturbatory Ideologies

Musturbatory Ideology 1: I *absolutely must* under all conditions do important tasks well and *must* be approved by significant others or else I am an inadequate and unlovable person.

Musturbatory Ideology 2: Other people *absolutely must* under all conditions treat me fairly and justly or else they are *rotten, damnable* people.

Musturbatory Ideology 3: Conditions under which I live *absolutely must* always be the way I want them to be, give me almost immediate gratification and not require me to work too hard to change or improve them, or else it is awful, I can't stand them, and it is impossible for me to be happy at all.

In his subsequent writings, Ellis has usually stuck to these three categories of irrational philosophies of life. In the third edition of the book, *A Guide to Rational Living*, which he co-authored with Dr Robert A. Harper (Ellis & Harper, 1997), there is a list of 10 irrational beliefs—a list that represents a revised version of his original list of 12. If we review this list carefully, we will realize that the above three musturbatory ideologies are prevalent in these beliefs as well. Let us see a few of the beliefs.

1. It is a dire necessity for an adult to be loved by everyone for everything he does. (Musturbatory Ideology 1)
2. Certain acts are wrong, wicked or villainous, and the people who perform such acts *should* be severely punished. (Musturbatory Ideology 2)
3. It is terrible, horrible and catastrophic when things are not the way one would like them to be. (Musturbatory Ideology 3)
4. Much human unhappiness is externally caused and is forced on one by outside people and events. (Musturbatory Ideology 2, 3)
5. If something is or may be dangerous or fearsome, one *should* be terribly concerned about it. (Musturbatory Ideology 3)

Ellis' further clinical experience brought to his attention that almost all human beings held all the three musturbatory ideologies, though in different proportions, and disturbed themselves at least to some extent.

Irrational Evaluative Beliefs and Derivatives

REBT proposes four types of irrational evaluative beliefs which are detrimental to mental health. Evaluative beliefs are people's abstractions about themselves, others or their lives. They are regarded as 'hot' cognitions fundamental to the arousal of self-defeating emotions.

Musturbatory ideology or demandingness is considered as the main type of evaluative belief. When a man held any one of these three musturbatory ideologies or philosophies of life, he also believed in three other evaluative beliefs which derive from the main belief.

Awfulizing: Awfulizing is a result of rating an observed adversity as being more than 100 per cent bad—an exaggerated conclusion that stems from the belief that 'this *must* not be as bad as it is'. In awfulizing, a person exaggerates the consequences and thinks that it is the worst thing that could happen. The people who awfulize often use terms such as horrible, terrible or awful.

I-can't-stand-it-itis: This means that a man cannot have any happiness if an observed adversity that *must* not happen actually happens and he cannot tolerate this circumstance or event. It is often referred to as 'discomfort tolerance'.

Damnation: This refers to a man's tendency to rate himself or others as 'subhuman' or 'undeserving' if he does something that he *must not* do or fails to do something that he *must* do. In damnation, a person rates self or someone else in totality on the basis of observation of specific trait or behaviour. Hence, it involves the tendency of overgeneralization. Finally, *damnation* also refers to a man's tendency to rate the conditions under which he lives (or even the world in which he lives) as being *rotten* for not granting him what he *must* have. This tendency leads to self-downing or other-downing, depression, grandiosity, etc.

According to Ellis, 'awfulizing', ' I-can't-stand-it- itis' and 'damnation' are secondary processes in the sense that they are derived from a man's musturbatory philosophy of life. For example, if a person has the belief that he *must* always succeed (Musturbatory Ideology 1), he is likely to get involved in awfulization by saying that it is awful for me to fail and if this happens, I can't stand it! (I-can't-stand-it- itis). And if I am not able to stand the failure, it shows that I am a worthless person (damnation).

However, Dr R.L. Wessler, (1984), a one-time close associate of Ellis, holds that they are often primary irrational philosophies of life and the musturbatory philosophies are derived from them. Perhaps, it is difficult to say which irrational philosophy is primary and which irrational philosophy is secondary. Dr Windy Dryden observes that they are two sides of the same cognitive coin (Neenan & Dryden, 2006).

The meaning of three primary musturbatory ideologies and the secondary beliefs derived from them will become clear if we apply them to the emotional disturbance of our three cases.

Analysis of Cases 5.1, 5.2 and 5.3 in Light of the Musturbatory Ideologies

Aditi: Aditi is feeling anxious because she thinks that her ignorance will be exposed if she goes to any interview. This obviously means that she is a victim of the *first musturbatory ideology* and therefore her belief about any interview is that 'I absolutely *must* do perfectly well in any interview and *must* be approved by people I consider significant or else I am an *inadequate and unlovable* person'.

The first derivative of her musturbatory ideology: 'It is "awful", meaning more than 100 per cent bad if my ignorance is exposed and I am disapproved by people I consider significant in my life'.

The second derivative of her musturbatory ideology: 'I cannot have any happiness in my life if my ignorance is exposed'.

Third derivative of her musturbatory ideology: 'If my ignorance is exposed, it will mean that I am a worthless, subhuman person who deserves nothing good in life'.

Vikram: Vikram is angry with his boss because he thinks that his boss *must* not use dictatorial methods of getting work done from him. This obviously means that he clings to the *second musturbatory ideology* and therefore his belief about his boss is that 'My boss absolutely *must* treat me fairly or justly or else he is a *rotten, damnable* person'.

The first derivative of his musturbatory ideology: 'It is "awful", meaning more than 100 per cent bad that my boss uses unfair and unjust methods of getting work done'.

The second derivative of his musturbatory ideology: 'I cannot have any happiness because my boss uses unfair and unjust methods of getting work done'.

The third derivative of his musturbatory ideology: 'As my boss uses unfair and unjust methods of getting work done from me, he is a worthless, subhuman person who deserves nothing good in life'.

Saniya: Saniya is feeling depressed because she thinks that the diet prescribed by her doctor *must* not be too hard to follow for a long time. This means that she is in the grip of the *third musturbatory ideology* and therefore her belief about the diet prescribed by the doctor is that 'The diet prescribed by the doctor *must not* require me to work too hard for a long time in order to improve my physical well-being'.

The first derivative of her musturbatory ideology: 'It is "awful", meaning more than 100 per cent bad that the diet prescribed by my doctor is too difficult to follow for a long time'.

The second derivative of her musturbatory ideology: 'As the diet prescribed by my doctor is so difficult to follow for a long time, I cannot have happiness in life'.

The third derivative of her musturbatory ideology: 'The conditions under which I live *must* give me a diet which is easy to follow for a long time and as those conditions don't give me what they *must*, they are *rotten*'.

Thus, according to REBT, when human beings remain devoted to the philosophy of *musturbation* and its derivatives, they make themselves emotionally upset. Some psychologists (Beck et al., 1979; Burns, 1980) pointed out that the thinking of emotionally disturbed people reveal many illogicalities or cognitive distortions. Some of the most important cognitive distortions easily observable in thinking of emotionally disturbed people mentioned by Ellis & Dryden (1997, pp. 15–16) are as follows:

1. *All-or-none thinking*—'If I fail at any important task, as I *must* not, I am a *total* failure and *completely* unlovable!'
2. *Jumping to conclusions and negative non sequiturs*—'Since they have seen me dismally fail, as I *should* not have done, they will view me as an incompetent worm'.
3. *Fortune-telling*—'Because they are laughing at me for failing, they know that I *should* have succeeded, and they will despise me forever'.
4. *Focusing on the negative*—'Because I *can't stand* things going wrong, as they *must* not, I can't see any good happening in my life'.
5. *Disqualifying the positive*—'When they compliment me on the good things I have done, they are only being kind to me and forgetting the foolish things that I *should* not have done'.
6. *Allness and neverness*—'Because conditions of living *ought* to be good and actually are so bad and so intolerable, they'll *always* be this way and I'll *never* have any happiness'.
7. *Labelling and overgeneralization*—'Because I *must* not fail at important work and have done so, I am a *complete* loser and failure!'
8. *Personalizing*—'Since I am acting far worse than I *should* act and they are laughing, I am sure they are only laughing at me, and that is *awful*!'
9. *Phonyism*—'When I don't do as well as I *ought* to do and they still praise and accept me, I am a real phony and will soon fall on my face and show them how despicable I am!'
10. *Perfectionism*—'I realize that I did fairly well, but I *should* have done perfectly well on a task like this and am therefore really an incompetent!'

Ellis concurs with the view that illogicalities such as those mentioned here characterize human emotional disturbance. He believed that such distortions in thinking are a result of the philosophy of *musturbation*, that is, they almost always stem from *musts*.

Desires and demands: REBT theory advocates the philosophy of 'desiring'. It states that humans have many desires, wishes, preferences, wants and so forth. Having these desires or wishes do not create emotional disturbance. On the contrary, emotionally healthy people do show desires. Desires give purpose and meaning to life. If we had no desires, we would hardly survive.

REBT encourages people to have strong and intense desires, wishes and preferences and to avoid feelings of detachment, withdrawal and lack of involvement (Ellis & Dryden, 1997). It states that human beings do not get disturbed if they have only desires in their mind. There is no reason why people *must* get what they desire. Realistically speaking, there is little relationship between what they desire and what they *must* get. Without considering this point, they irrationally believe that their desires *must* be satisfied. REBT proposes that when people escalate their desires into dogmatic demands, they get emotionally disturbed. For example, in Aditi's case, if she states that 'I really want to do well in the interview', she will not get disturbed as she is expressing only desire. However, she doesn't stop at the desire and says that 'because I really want to do well in the interview, therefore I *absolutely have* to do so'. Now she added dogmatic demand into her desire, which takes her towards and therefore is disturbed.

A REBT therapist helps people to differentiate between dogmatic demands and desires and teach them how to surrender the former and retain the latter. He will show them that if people have only desires, and if these desires are not fulfilled, they will experience healthy negative emotions such as sadness, irritation, regret, frustration and disappointment. These emotions are constructive and help people to achieve their goals. We will see the detailed description of these emotions in the later part of this chapter.

Absolutistic *Musts/Shoulds*

We have seen that dogmatic *musts* or demands stay at the core of psychological disturbance. These dogmatic *musts* are called *absolutistic demands*. REBT makes a clear distinction between absolute and non-absolute *shoulds* or *musts*. Absolutistic *shoulds* or *musts* lead to emotional disturbance whereas conditional *musts* and *shoulds* do not cause disturbance. In this context, it is necessary to know different ways of using the word '*should*' in the English language. A list of these *shoulds* is described in the *Training Handbook of the Fundamentals of REBT* (Dryden & Branch, 2008).

Recommendatory *should*: This '*should*' specifies a recommendation for self or other, for example, 'You *should* read this book' translates to 'I recommend that you read this book' or 'I really *should* go to bed early tonight' means 'It's in my best interest to go to bed early tonight'.

Predictive *should*: This use of '*should*' indicates predictions about the future, for example, 'I *should* be on time for my flight' is interpreted as 'I predict that I will be on time for my flight'.

Ideal *Should*: This '*should*' describes ideal conditions, for example, 'People *should* not litter' expresses the viewpoint 'ideally, people *should* not litter'.

Empirical *should*: This '*should*' points to the existence of reality. It encapsulates the idea that an event *should* occur when all conditions are in place for it. For example, 'The car *should* have broken down because it is old and in ill repair' or 'You *should* have fallen when you stepped off the ladder because of the laws of gravity'.

Preferential *should*: This '*should*' indicates a desire or preference for a given condition to exist, for example, 'My husband *should* preferably remember our anniversary' carries an implicit additional meaning that 'it would be good if he remembered but he does not have to'.

Conditional *should/must*: This '*should*' denotes that in order for one condition to exist, another primary condition *must* be met. For example, 'I *should* eat healthily in order to become slimmer' and 'I *must* pass the interview in order to be accepted onto the course'.

Absolutistic *should*: This term obviously refers to the disturbance-creating demands at B in the ABC model of REBT. 'I absolutely *should* visit my aunt in the hospital' and 'I absolutely *must* tend to my aunt at all times and under any conditions' are examples of absolute *shoulds*.

REBT holds the view that these meanings of *should* except absolutistic *should/must* will not create emotional disturbance. Absolutistic *should* is dogmatic or rigid in the form. For example, when Aditi says 'because I really want to do well in the interview, therefore I *absolutely have to* do so', her demand is irrational for the following reasons:

- Aditi does not allow for the fact that she might not do well. It is inconsistent with reality as it assumes that if there is a law of the universe that compels Aditi to *must* do well in the interview. If this law really exists, then there would be no possibility that she would not perform well in it. Obviously, no such law exists.

- It is illogical as there is no logical connection between her desire that she wants to do well which is not rigid and her absolutistic demand that she *absolutely has* to do so, which is rigid. In logic, something rigid cannot logically follow from something that is not rigid.
- It leads to unhealthy emotions of anxiety and dysfunctional behaviour of avoidance to go for an interview. This interferes with her persuasion of a long-term goal of getting a good job. It interferes with her doing well, that is, the absolutistic demand draws her to focus on how she *should* not go wrong rather than how she can prepare for the interview.

This is not to say that absolutistic thinking always leads to poor results. Sometimes it motivates people to achieve their goals. That is why absolutistic thinking gets reinforced and become quite vehement in their mind. However, if we carefully observe, this thinking will help them only in short-term achievements. In the long run, it leads to dysfunctional emotions and behaviour. For example, if the child says that 'I *have to absolutely* get the first rank in class', it is possible that the child gets motivated due to this absolutistic thinking and strives hard to get the first rank. Outwardly, it appears that absolutistic thinking is helping him achieve his goal, but in reality, it creates long-term harm to his mental health. Since he has achieved his goal successfully, he now thinks that in order to achieve his goal, he needs to think in absolutistic terms. Hence, he will use this thinking predominantly for every goal attainment. His absolutistic thinking does not give him a scope to accept the fact that he might not stand first in every exam. As a result of this, when he does not stand first in any exam, he pays the huge cost of emotional disturbance. He might lose his confidence and go into depression. In the long run, there is a high probability that absolutistic thinking sabotages the mental health of people and creates obstruction in their goal attainment.

Biological Basis of Irrational Thinking

When Ellis created REBT in 1955, he was by and large an environmentalist and believed that significant events in man's life play an important role in psychological disturbance. However, his reading and clinical experience made him revise this view.

In 1976, he published a paper titled 'The Biological Basis of Human Irrationality' in the *Journal of Individual Psychology* (Ellis, 1976). In this paper, he stressed that irrational thinking which causes emotional disturbance is mainly determined by biological factors, although those factors always interact with significant environmental conditions. According to him, even if a human being is lucky to have very sensible, rational parents and other family members, he would turn his wants and preferences to absolutistic *musts, shoulds and oughts*. He gave many observations supporting his hypothesis. Some of them are as follows:

1. Even the most intelligent human beings think irrationally.
2. Almost all irrationalities which create emotional disturbance are noticed in all societies and cultures.
3. Human beings procrastinate and lack self-discipline in spite of the teaching of their parents, peers, teachers, etc.
4. If a man gives up one form of irrationality, he falls prey to some other form of irrationality.
5. If a man strongly opposes some kind of irrationality, he sometimes becomes a devout believer in that very irrationality. For instance, some people who strongly deny the existence of God subsequently become devotedly religious.
6. The knowledge of how excessive alcohol consumption is injurious to his health and life does not prevent a man from drinking it in large quantities.
7. A man may work very hard to overcome some of his handicapping habits and behaviour patterns but finally returns to them again.
8. Human beings find it easy to learn self-defeating activities than self-enhancing ones. They find it very easy to overeat, but they find it very difficult to eat moderately.
9. Therapists also behave irrationally in their own lives.
10. Many people manage to convince themselves that certain bad events such as accidents, illness, etc. will not happen in their lives.

These and similar observations may support Ellis's hypothesis that human beings are born with a biological tendency to think irrationally. However, Ellis mentioned that in addition to irrational thinking, a man has a biological tendency to think rationally as well. In fact, he believed that there are two fundamental biological tendencies of man. One of them is to think irrationally and the second one is, of course, to think rationally and to work hard at changing his irrational thinking. Thus, he optimistically believes that man has the ability to overcome, at least to a certain extent, his biological tendency to think irrationally.

Yet it needs to be mentioned that Ellis was often strongly criticized for upholding that biological factors contribute to human irrationality. Many critics raised the objection that if man's biological inheritance plays considerable part in human personality, there will be no role left for psychotherapists to bring desirable changes in him. However, this fear is baseless. Such changes can be brought about by recognizing that the task is difficult, not impossible.

Inferences, Evaluations and Core Beliefs

Froggatt (2005) proposed three levels of thinking as inferences, evaluations and beliefs.

1. **Inferences:** This thinking goes beyond the available data and includes some predictions. They can be true or false. For example, it is raining heavily and it will continue to rain for the next few hours. These inferences are non-evaluative when they are not related to our goal. If they are related to our goal, they become evaluative. For example, it is raining heavily and if it continues to rain for next few hours, it will be inconvenient for me to drive.

   In REBT, little attention is given to inferences as they are non-evaluative in nature.

2. **Evaluations:** REBT focuses more on evaluations as they go beyond the available data and are related to our goal. We evaluate the activating event in terms of what it means to us. We attach some value to it or make judgements. Evaluations can be rational or irrational.

Ellis and Dryden (1997) classified these evaluations in four different types.

(i) *Positive preferential evaluations (rational)*—These evaluations are non-absolute wishes, expectations or desires. They include positive evaluations about the activating event. They are regarded as rational in REBT. For example, 'I wish to succeed in my endeavour'.

(ii) *Positive musturbatory evaluations (irrational)*—These evaluations consist of absolutistic and dogmatic demands. They include unrealistic positive evaluations of the activating event. They are termed irrational. For example, 'I *must* succeed in my endeavour or I am sure I will succeed in my endeavour'.

(iii) *Negative preferential evaluations (rational)*—These evaluations are flexible and non-absolute. They include negative evaluations of the activating event. These evaluations are considered rational. For example, 'It is difficult to bear if I fail in the endeavour'.

(iv) *Negative musturbatory evaluations (irrational)*—These evaluations are absolutistic and dogmatic in nature. They include unrealistic negative evaluations of the activating event. These evaluations are considered irrational. For example, 'It is unbearable to me if I fail in the endeavour'.

3. **Core beliefs:** Guiding a person's inferences and evaluations are their underlying general core beliefs. Core beliefs can be rational or irrational. The beliefs that are based on irrational evaluations are called irrational evaluative beliefs, which are listed earlier.

More About Consequences

We shall now focus our attention to 'C' in the ABC theory. Roughly speaking, the letter C stands for the emotional consequences that a man experiences as a result of an Adversity (A) he faces in his life and his Belief (B) about it.

Analysis of Cases 5.1, 5.2 and 5.3 in Light of the Consequences

Let us review the emotional disturbance of these three cases. Aditi, Vikram and Saniya are suffering from anxiety, anger and depression respectively. Or to put it in terms of the ABC theory, Aditi, Vikram and Saniya are experiencing the consequences (C) of anxiety, anger and depression, respectively. A careful study of the problems faced by them reveals the complexity of their emotional disturbances.

Emotional, physiological and behavioural consequences: Aditi feels anxiety about going for the interview (emotional). Her anxiety is accompanied by avoidance to go for the interview (behavioural). Apart from this, thinking about the interview causes her head to ache (physiological).

Vikram is angry with his boss (emotional). His anger is accompanied by his dodging work every morning and also behaving in a hostile manner (behavioural). He experiences rapid heart rate and feels hot in his body, when he thinks of his boss (physiological). Saniya is not only feeling depressed (emotional) but is also not following the diet recommended to her by doctor (behavioural). This causes her to feel tired and exhausted (physiological). This means that at point C, they not only experience a certain emotion but experience some physiological symptoms as well. They act or behave in a certain manner. Therefore, in the ABC theory, the letter C denotes emotional, physiological and behavioural consequences.

Multiplicity of Consequences

We shall return to our three cases and reconsider their specific emotional and behavioural problems caused by the individual musturbatory ideology that each of them is holding.

Aditi: Aditi is experiencing anxiety and headache, and is also avoiding to go to the job interview for which she has received a call. These emotional, physiological and behavioural consequences are largely created by her belief in Musturbatory Ideology 1, which in essence means demanding perfection of oneself.

This is a gross oversimplification of Aditi's emotional, physiological and behavioural disturbance. Her firm belief in this musturbatory ideology may create more emotional, physiological and behavioural handicaps, if she interprets and evaluates her past experiences of feeling anxious, having headaches and avoiding interviews. As a result of this and the other mental activities, she may create emotional consequences of depression, despair and feeling of worthlessness or self-damnation. Along with these emotional consequences, she may exhibit physiological consequences such as severe pain in the head and behavioural consequences of avoidance, withdrawal and even addiction.

Aditi may bring to the therapist some other emotional, physiological and behavioural problems if she is clinging to the second and third musturbatory ideologies, along with the first one. As a matter of fact, a human being is rarely afflicted with only one *must*. For the most part of his life, he is a victim of all three *musts*, although in different degrees.

Vikram: Vikram is angry with his boss, has a rapid heart rate, feels hot in his body and shows reluctance to go to work every morning. These emotional, physiological and behavioural consequences are largely created by his belief in the second musturbatory ideology, the essence of which lies in demanding perfection of others.

However, Vikram's emotional, physiological and behavioural problems can be more complex. In accordance with his strong belief in this musturbatory ideology, he may create more emotional, physiological and behavioural difficulties for everyone (including himself). He obsessively broods over and evaluates his boss method of getting work done for a long time. For instance, he may become a victim of self-created emotional consequences of rage, furry, resentment and even revenge. These emotions may give rise to increased physiological symptoms such as high blood pressure, muscle tension, palpitation and also several behavioural consequences including hostile verbal exchanges with his boss and instigating other employees to disobey the boss' instructions. When some people are inflamed with resentment and revenge, they behave in many violent ways.

Besides, people who embrace the second musturbatory ideology can also embrace the first one and the third one as well. In that case, they may bring to the therapist some other emotional, physiological and behavioural problems.

Saniya: Saniya is beset with the problem of rigorously following the special diet prescribed by her doctor. She feels depressed, exhausted and has given up on the goal of reducing her weight by 5 kg. These emotional, physiological and behavioural consequences are largely a product of her whole-hearted acceptance of Musturbatory Ideology 3, which consists of demanding that conditions in the world be easy.

Saniya may be faced with even more emotional, physiological and behavioural problems. Her staunch belief in this musturbatory ideology can give rise to emotional consequences such as rage, rebellion, low frustration tolerance (LFT) and self-pity and physiological consequences such as sleep disturbances or gastrointestinal problems. As a result, she may exhibit the behavioural consequences of withdrawal, procrastination, inertia and even addiction.

Saniya may bring to the therapist, additional emotional, physiological and behavioural problems if she also holds the second and third musturbatory ideologies. It is necessary to reiterate this because of his biosocial makeup that a human being is prone to believe in all the three musturbatory ideologies; although, the proportion of those beliefs varies considerably from person to person.

Disturbance about Disturbance

Primary disturbance: Soon after Ellis began to use REBT on his clients, he could see that many of his clients were disturbing themselves emotionally about their main disturbance (primary disturbance in terms of REBT). For instance, if a client was feeling anxious about taking an examination in his college, Ellis found it easy to interpret his anxiety according to the ABC theory. Obviously, the prospect of appearing for a certain examination was an Activating event or Adversity (A) in the client's life. His demand that he *should* do well in that examination (Musturbatory Ideology 1) was his Belief (B) and his anxiety was largely a self-created emotional Consequence (C) in his mind.

Secondary disturbance: The anxiety mentioned previously was his primary disturbance. Due to the client's biosocial tendency to observe and evaluate practically everything in his life, he observed his primary disturbance or primary symptom, and that observation itself became a new Activating event or Adversity in his life. Further, because he interpreted and evaluated his primary symptom of anxiety in the light of his Belief (B) that he *must* be in perfect control of himself and therefore *must* never feel anxious, he created the emotional consequences of depression and guilt in his mind. Thus, he created a secondary emotional disturbance about his primary emotional disturbance or symptom. In other words, he developed 'symptom-stress' in his mind. Or he created a secondary emotional disturbance. Similarly, it is not unrealistic to expect that our three cases—Aditi, Vikram and Saniya—may disturb themselves over their primary disturbances.

Analysis of Cases 5.1, 5.2 and 5.3 in the Light of Primary and Secondary Disturbance

Aditi: Perhaps, this is how Aditi can disturb herself about her primary emotional disturbance, namely, anxiety. She is anxious about going for the job interview. When she notices that she is anxious, her very primary symptom of anxiety becomes a new Activating Event or Adversity in her life. She will then interpret and evaluate that anxiety according to the peculiar set of musturbatory ideologies she subscribes to, thereby creating a secondary emotional disturbance of depression, guilt and self-pity in her mind.

Vikram: Vikram's primary emotional disturbance is anger towards his boss. As he observes that he is angry with his boss, his very primary emotional disturbance of anger becomes a new activating event or adversity in his life. He will then interpret and evaluate that anger in his mind in accordance with the peculiar set of musturbatory ideologies he holds and thereby creates a secondary emotional disturbance of self-hatred, guilt, and shame in his mind.

Saniya: Saniya's primary emotional disturbance is depression at the prospect of rigorously implementing the special diet prescribed by her doctor. When she becomes aware of her primary emotional disturbance, that awareness itself can become a new Activating event or Adversity in her life. Then, guided by the peculiar mix of musturbatory ideologies she adheres to, she will interpret and evaluate her depression and thereby create in her mind a secondary emotional disturbance of shame, guilt, self-loathing and even depression about her depression.

In a nutshell, it may be said that any primary emotional disturbance can give rise to a new cycle of $A \times B = C$, creating a secondary emotional disturbance. In this way, a disturbed client can disturb himself about his disturbance itself. Sometimes, this kind of a cycle can lead to even a tertiary disturbance because any secondary emotional disturbance can serve as still another Activating event or Adversity in the client's life. Governed by his peculiar combination of musturbatory ideologies, the client interprets and evaluates a new Activating Event or Adversity which, in turn, leads to the creation of a tertiary disturbance in his mind.

All this means that an emotional disturbance is a complex matter as it can give rise to a chain of emotional disturbances.

Healthy and Unhealthy Emotions

From the foregoing discussion, it may be tempting to guess that the goal of REBT is to help emotionally disturbed people develop all positive emotions and to get rid of their all negative emotions. It is imperative to note that this is not exactly what REBT aims at. There are two issues involved here. We will first discuss the positive emotions and will then move on to the negative emotions.

Realistically positive: REBT is sometimes misunderstood as a promoter of positive thinking. There are many thinkers, such as, Emile Coue, Norman Vincent Peale, Maxwell Maltz, Napoleaon Hill and others, who advocate 'positive thinking'. They claim that positive thinkers are less neurotic and less disturbed than negative thinkers. They make positive affirmations such as 'day-by-day, in every way, I am getting better and better' or 'I am valuable and worthwhile' and so forth.

REBT differs from positive thinking in advocating 'realistic positive view' rather than merely 'accentuating the positive'. It says that a positive perspective is beneficial, provided that it is realistic. If we look at the world only through a positive lens, we tend to deny the existence of negative things, which is inconsistent with reality. REBT advocates that we look at the world realistically rather than only positively. A realistic outlook helps people maintain a positive perspective within the constraints of reality. A REBT therapist tries to show their clients that they may feel better due to 'positive thinking', but it will not help them thoroughly or permanently.

We will take Aditi's example to explain this point further. If Aditi has adopted positive thinking, she will positively affirm that her interview will go well. By this affirmation, there is a possibility that she may feel better for some time. However, in the long term, this will not be helpful for her in two ways. First, this thinking will prevent her from preparing for the interview. Since she is so confident about her good interview, she will not bother to prepare for it. It will sabotage her long-term goal of getting a good job. Second, this thinking is unrealistic. She does not have the facts to prove that her interview will surely go well. If it does not go well in reality, she will plunge into a storm of high emotional disturbance.

An REBT therapist will help her think realistically positive. She will prepare for her interview with a positive outlook but at the same time, will not deny the possibility of her interview not going well. She will not consider the latter as awful and will keep herself from getting disturbed.

In this context, REBT suggests that not all positive emotions are necessarily healthy. For example, the emotion of grandiosity. Though this emotion is positive, it presents an unrealistic evaluation about oneself. The person experiencing this emotion will not be ready to accept any negative evaluation about himself or herself and will get emotionally disturbed. REBT helps people get rid of unhealthy positive emotions. At the same time, it encourages healthy positive emotions including love, happiness, pleasure and curiosity.

Healthy negative emotions: Just as not all positive emotions are necessarily healthy, similarly not all negative emotions are necessarily unhealthy. REBT does not aim at helping upset people free themselves from all negative emotions and experience some sort of serenity.

Suppose a student's goal is to pass a certain examination, but he fails. Now how do we realistically expect him to feel? Is it realistic to expect him to feel happy about his failure? Is it realistic to expect that he experience profound serenity because of his failure? Besides, will happiness and serenity help him achieve his goal of passing that examination by appearing for it again?

REBT acknowledges that negative emotions have a rightful place in human life. When human beings do not achieve their goals, it is neither realistic nor useful for them to experience happiness, serenity or neutrality. On the contrary, it is realistic that they experience some negative emotion. In fact, negative emotions can spur them to go back to their goals and make efforts to realize those goals.

REBT makes a distinction between negative emotions that are potentially self-helpful (and therefore healthy) and negative emotions that are potentially self-defeating (and therefore unhealthy). For instance, a student who fails a certain examination allows himself to be overwhelmed by the feeling of depression and despair may abandon his goal itself. However, if he feels frustrated because of his failure (which is quite realistic), he may find out the probable cause and then reappear for that examination with renewed determination and hope. That means that initially experiencing the negative emotion of frustration can prove self-helping to him in the long run. Therefore, REBT regards the negative emotion of frustration as a potentially self-helping and healthy emotion. It regards the negative emotions of depression and despair as potentially self-defeating and unhealthy emotions. Naturally, it is not the aim of REBT to help people get rid of all negative emotions. It encourages healthy negative emotions that include concern, annoyance, regret, disappointment and frustration.

From this description, it is clear why Ellis had not chosen to classify emotions as positive or negative. He had instead categorized them under two headings—healthy and unhealthy. Table 6.1 presents a list of the major healthy and unhealthy negative emotions as described by Ellis. Table 6.1 shows major healthy emotions on the left side and their unhealthy counterparts on the right side.

Table 6.1

Classification of Healthy and Unhealthy Emotions

Healthy Emotions	Unhealthy Emotions
Concern	Anxiety
Sadness	Depression
Annoyance	Anger
Regret	Guilt
Disappointment	Shame
Frustration	Self-pity

Source: Yankura and Dryden (1994).

Concern versus anxiety: A concerned person believes, 'I wish that the adversity does not occur. However, if it occurs, it would be unpleasant but not awful'. An anxious person believes that 'the adversity *must* not occur and it would be *awful* it does. I *can't stand* this awful situation'. Concern consists of the objective evaluation of the situation whereas anxiety consists of the unrealistic evaluation of the situation and oneself. Concern is healthy as it motivates the person to take constructive action towards the adverse situation. In anxiety, instead of taking constructive action, the person focuses on the unrealistic evaluation of his performance in the situation.

Sadness versus depression: In sadness, the person believes, 'Something which I do not want has happened, but there is no reason why it *should* not have happened'. In depression, on the other hand, the person believes, 'This situation *should* not have occurred and it is so *terrible* that I will *never* cope with it'. Sadness is healthy as it provokes the person to search for the causes of the unfortunate situation and take corrective actions if possible. Depression on the other hand is unhealthy as the person jumps on the unrealistic conclusions about the future and becomes inactive.

Annoyance versus anger: In annoyance, the person believes, 'I don't like what he did. It would be better if he had not done so. There is no reason to believe that he *must* have done so'. In anger, the person believes that other absolutely *must* not do that act and thus *damns* the other for doing so. An annoyed person does not like what the other has done but does not damn him or her for doing it. Annoyance is healthy as it focuses on others' *act* but not at the *person* for acting badly. Anger is unhealthy as the person unrealistically concludes that other person will act similarly in future situations too and therefore closes the option that he might act differently in different situation.

Regret versus guilt: Regret occurs when a person acknowledges that he has done something that he is not supposed to do. He feels bad about the act but accepts himself as a fallible human being for doing so. He takes precaution not to repeat the behaviour in the future. In guilt, the person damns himself as bad, wicked or rotten for acting badly. He says, 'I *must* not act badly, and if I act, it's *awful* and I am a *rotten* person!' Regret is healthy as it focuses on *act* and allows improvement but guilt focuses on person and therefore denies the opportunity for improvement.

Disappointment versus shame: When the person does a stupid act in front of others, he may feel either disappointment or shame. In disappointment, the person acknowledges the stupid act (without labelling himself) even if people think badly about him. In shame, the person believes that other people are thinking badly about him due to his stupid act and that it is *horrible* and therefore condemns himself for acting stupidly in public, something that he *should* not have done. Disappointment is healthy as the person evaluates his act and does not need the approval of others, whereas shame is unhealthy as it involves self-denigration and the *absolutistic* need of approval from others.

Frustration versus self-pity: In frustration, the person believes, 'It is a tough task. There is a barrier between my efforts and the goal to be attained. How can I improve my efforts, to remove the barrier?' In self-pity, the person believes, 'I am destined to get obstacles in my goal attainment. Even if I work hard, I will not able to reach the goal due to my poor destiny'. Frustration is healthy as it motivates the person to find out various ways to achieve the goal. Self-pity is unhealthy as the person is unrealistically convinced about his failure in goal attainment and therefore divers away from goal.

To summarize, REBT encourages person's negative healthy emotion as they are deemed to be consequences of rational thinking. Therapeutic change is needed for people who show negative unhealthy emotions.

Qualitative difference: A very important point to be noted about healthy and unhealthy negative emotions is that unhealthy negative emotions are not just intense versions of healthy negative emotions. For example, the negative emotion of self-pity is not just an intense version of the negative emotion of frustration. On the contrary, frustration and self-pity are qualitatively different emotions because they arise out of different beliefs. Frustration is a result of viewing an obstacle in one's path from the standpoint of a rational belief, that is, the philosophy of wanting something. Self-pity is a result of viewing an obstacle in one's path from the standpoint of an irrational belief, that is, the philosophy of demanding something. However, though emotions of frustration and self-pity are qualitatively different because they arise from different beliefs or philosophies of life, both of them can be mild, moderate or intense. Now let us consider whether the negative emotions of our three cases are self-helping and healthy.

Analysis of Cases 5.1, 5.2 and 5.3 in Light of Healthy and Unhealthy Emotions

Aditi: The cause of Aditi's anxiety is her adherence to Musturbatory Ideology 1 which demands perfection of oneself. Her anxiety is not helping her to go for the job interview. Therefore, her negative emotion of anxiety is to be considered as a self-defeating, unhealthy negative emotion. On the contrary, if she looks at her goal of getting a job from the standpoint of a rational belief and then fails to achieve it, she may create the self-helping, healthy negative emotion of concern in her mind. She may then determinedly go for the job interview.

Vikram: Vikram creates anger in his mind because he is clung to Musturbatory Ideology 2 which demands the kind and just behaviour of others, especially his boss. His anger is definitely not helping him to come to terms with his boss. As a matter of fact, his anger is making him reluctant about going to work everyday morning. His negative emotion of anger is to be regarded as a self-defeating and unhealthy negative emotion. If he looks at his goal of continuing to hold his job at least for a year from the standpoint of a rational belief, he may create the self-helping, healthy negative emotion of annoyance in his mind in case his goal is not realized. This emotion may help him find out ways and means of coping with his boss' methods of getting work done from his subordinates without unnecessarily harming himself.

Saniya: Saniya is in the grip of depression because she devoutly subscribes to Musturbatory Ideology 3 which demands ease and comfort of the environment or conditions around her. However, depression is certainly not helping her to rigorously follow the special diet prescribed by her doctor. In view of this, her negative emotion of depression is to be categorized as a self-defeating, unhealthy negative emotion. Whereas, if she gives up her absolutistic demand for an easy-to-follow special diet and instead asks for it, she may create a self-helping, healthy negative emotion of frustration in her mind if her desire or preference is unfulfilled. This emotion may help her to find out ways and means of persistently following the special diet prescribed by her doctor.

Relationship between beliefs and emotions: The description in the preceding section leads to the logical question: If according to the ABC theory, consequences are largely caused by beliefs, which beliefs give rise to potentially self-helping and healthy negative emotions, and which beliefs give rise to potentially self-defeating and unhealthy negative emotions? The answer to this question is simple. That answer is all musturbatory ideologies lead to potentially self-defeating unhealthy negative emotions. The chief characteristic of all musturbatory ideologies is that they turn human desires, wants and expectations into inflexible demands, commands and *musts*. A student who adheres to Musturbatory Ideology 1, which in essence means that he *must* pass a certain examination, is likely to become anxious or even panicky before that examination and also create feelings of depression and despair in his mind if he fails to achieve his goal. On the contrary, a student who wants (or even intensely wants) to pass a certain examination is likely to experience concern (or even intense concern) before that examination and create frustration (and even intense frustration) in his mind if he fails to achieve his goal.

Thus, one of the cardinal principle of REBT is that when human beings turn their desires into demands, they are likely to create self-defeating and unhealthy negative emotions in their minds. In other words, when they hold rational, reasonable, realistic and flexible beliefs about their goals, they are likely to experience self-helping and healthy negative emotions in case they fail to fulfil their goals, desires, wants and expectations. On the contrary, when they hold irrational, unreasonable, unrealistic and inflexible beliefs about their goals, they become prone to create self-defeating and unhealthy negative emotions in their minds.

So much for the appropriateness and usefulness of negative emotions in human life! As the three musturbatory ideologies give rise to different self-defeating, unhealthy negative emotions, it would be useful to get acquainted with a few other emotions in this category and their corresponding self-helping, healthy negative counterparts.

Musturbatory Ideology 1: The essence of this ideology is demanding perfection of oneself. Therefore, it is a potential source of self-defeating, unhealthy negative emotions such as anxiety and even panic, shame or embarrassment, guilt, irrational or senseless jealousy, etc. Whereas, if this philosophy of demanding is turned into a philosophy of desiring or preferring, it becomes a potential source of self-helping, healthy negative emotions such as concern, disappointment, regret and rational or sensible jealousy.

Musturbatory Ideology 2: The gist of this ideology is demanding kind and just behaviour of others. Therefore, it is a potential source of self-defeating, unhealthy negative emotions such as anger, rage, hatred and revenge. However, if this philosophy of demanding is turned into a philosophy of expecting kind and just behaviour of others, it becomes a potential source of self-helping, healthy negative emotions of annoyance or irritation.

Musturbatory Ideology 3: The core of this ideology consists of demanding ease and comfort of the environmental conditions in the world. Naturally, it becomes a potential source of self-defeating, negative emotions such as depression, helplessness and self-pity. However, if this philosophy of demanding is turned into a philosophy of wishing to live under easy and comfortable conditions, it becomes a potential source of self-helping healthy negative emotions such as frustration, sadness, etc.

Two Types of Anxiety

By now, it is clear that human beings disturb themselves emotionally when they subscribe to the philosophy of demandingness or what Ellis calls *musturbation*. This demandingness can be directed at oneself, others and the existing conditions.

Ego anxiety: However, Ellis' growing clinical experience made him aware that the three musturbatory ideologies could give rise to two types of anxiety. He called the first type of anxiety as 'ego anxiety'. Ego anxiety arises due to the absolutistic demands a person makes on self, others and the world. These demands are mostly perfectionist demands and, if they are not met in the past, present or future, the person gets disturbed by *damning self*. Self damnation involves (a) the process of giving myself a global negative rating and (b) 'devilifying' my 'self' as being bad or less worthy (Dryden, 1984).

Discomfort anxiety: The second type of anxiety is called as discomfort anxiety. It is also called LFT. This anxiety arises due to the absolutistic demands a person makes on self, others and the world. These demands are about the comfort that the world *must* be easy and comfortable. If these demands are not met in the past, present or future, a person gets disturbed and tends to *awfulize* and create I-can't-stand-it- itis.

Analysis of Cases 5.1, 5.2 and 5.3 in Light of the Types of Anxiety

Aditi: It is easy to understand the meaning of ego anxiety by reviewing Aditi's emotional disturbance. As she is overwhelmed by Musturbatory Ideology 1, she demands that she *must* do perfectly well in the job interview and earn the appreciation of significant people in her life; or else, she will be *worthless*. Thus, she stakes her ego on the job interview and thereby creates what is called ego anxiety in her mind.

Aditi also makes herself anxious because she thinks she will experience *intolerable discomfort* if her demand is not met. As per Ellis, this second anxiety faced by Aditi is called discomfort anxiety.

Vikram: As Vikram is clinging to Musturbatory Ideology 2, he demands that his boss *must* use just and kind methods of getting work done. Hence, he is angry with his boss. Vikram's attitude towards himself makes him think that he is *worthless* if his boss does not treat him justly and kindly. This creates ego anxiety in his mind.

At the same time, Vikram also believes that he *cannot stand* life conditions if his boss does not treat him justly and kindly. This creates discomfort anxiety in his mind as well.

Saniya: Saniya adheres to Musturbatory Ideology 3, and therefore by demanding that she *must* find the special diet prescribed by her doctor easy to follow, she makes herself a victim of ego anxiety.

Saniya also believes that if the special diet prescribed by her doctor is not easy to follow, she will experience *intolerable* distress. This belief gives rise to discomfort anxiety in her mind.

The prevalence of these two types of anxiety is so widespread among the emotionally disturbed clients that REBT presumes that most clients are afflicted with both kinds of anxieties.

This was about the letter C (consequences) of the ABC theory of emotional disturbance. With this elaboration of all the three letters, we have covered almost all the significant features of this theory. One may expect that the next topic will be therapeutic process and techniques used in REBT. However, it may be recalled that yet another important component of REBT is the philosophy of life. It is time to address that component. The process and techniques of REBT will be reviewed thereafter.

References

Beck, A.T., Rush, A.J. Shaw, B.F., & Emery, G. (1979). *Cognitive Therapy of Depression.* New York, NY: Guilford.

Burns, D.D. (1980). *Feeling Good: The New Mood Therapy.* New York, NY: Morrow.

Dryden, W. (1984). Rational-emotive therapy. In W. Dryden (Eds), *Individual Therapy in Britain* (pp. 235–63). London: Harper & Row.

Dryden, W., & Branch, R. (2008). *The Fundamentals of Rational Emotive Behaviour Therapy: A Training Handbook* (2nd edition, pp. 15–16). West Sussex: John Wiley & Sons.

Ellis, A. (1976). The biological basis of human irrationality. *Journal of Individual Psychology, 32* (November, 2): 145–68.

Ellis, A., & Dryden, W. (1997). *The Practice of Rational-Emotive Therapy* (2nd edition, pp. 7, 9–12, 15–16, 20). New York, NY: Springer.

Ellis, A., & Harper, R. A. (1997). *A Guide to Rational Living.* (3rd rev. ed.). Modesto, CA: Melvin Powers.

Froggatt, W. (2005). *A Brief Introduction to Cognitive-Behaviour Therapy* (3rd ed.). Retrieved from www.rational.org.nz/prof-docs/Intro-CBT.pdf

Neenan, M., & Dryden W. (2006) *Rational Emotive Behaviour Therapy in a Nutshell* (1st edition, p. 13). Thousand Oaks, CA: SAGE.

Wessler, R.L. (1984). Alternative conceptions of rational-emotive therapy: Toward a philosophically neutral psychotherapy. In M.A. Reda & M.J. Mahoney (Eds.), *Cognitive Psychotherapies: Recent Developments in Theory, Research and Practice* (pp. 65–79). Cambridge, MA: Ballinger.

Yankura, J., & Dryden, W. (1994). *Albert Ellis* (p. 34). Key Figures in Counselling and Psychotherapy Series. London: SAGE Publications.

Further Readings

Ellis, A. (1962). *Reason and Emotion in Psychotherapy*. New York, NY: Lyle Stuart. (Revised and updated edition, 1994). New York: Kensington Publishers.

———. (2001). *Feeling Better, Getting Better, Staying Better*. Atascadero, CA: Impact Publishers.

———. (1973). *How to Stubbornly Refuse to Be Ashamed of Anything*. Cassette Recording. New York, NY: Albert Ellis Institute.

Phadke, K.M. (1999). *Adhunik Sanjivani*. Mumbai: Tridal Prakashan.

7

REBT: Philosophy of Life

Ellis once commented that although he invented REBT in 1955, he was convinced at least 20 years before that if humans adapt a healthy philosophy of life, they will stay away from dysfunctional thoughts, emotions and behaviour. He further added that without this conviction, he would not have invented REBT (Phadke, 1968–2003).

This is literally true. Although Ellis held a doctorate in clinical psychology, since the age of 16, his pass-time had been philosophy and literature. He had always been keenly interested in the philosophy of human happiness. Just a few years after practising psychoanalysis, in which he had received systematic training, he became disillusioned with its theory and practice. One of his major charges against psychoanalysis was that it focuses too much on the historical details of clients' lives and overlooks the irrational philosophies which underpin their emotional disturbances.

After Ellis abandoned psychoanalysis, he began to search for the causes of his clients' emotional disturbances in their currently held faulty philosophies rather than their childhood experiences. In fact, he often said that a large part of REBT theory is derived from philosophy rather than psychology (Ellis, 1999, 2010).

He was by no means a stray wandering psychotherapist looking for the philosophical causes of emotional disturbances. He pointed out that Peter A. Bertocci (1963), in reviewing the work of Isdior Chein and Gordon Allport, mentioned about their realization that a psychology of personality is at the same time a philosophy of personality. Similarly, Mildred Newman and Bernard Berkowitz (1971) in their book, *How to Be Your Own Best Friend*, propagate a clear-cut philosophic approach to solving emotional problems. Philosophical approaches of Viktor Frankl (1959) and Rollo May (1967) are too pronounced to be neglected.

Hence, Ellis was not the only mental health professional who emphasized the philosophical roots of man's emotional disturbance. He not only emphasized but also offered some salient philosophical features as a vital component of REBT. A description of some of those features is provided here. From that, a mosaic of REBT's philosophy of life will gradually emerge.

REBT on Religion and Atheism

Dispute Over the Word 'Rational'

Since its inception, REBT, being rebellious, has met with opposition for many reasons. One of those reasons is the very name of its systems, namely, rational therapy, as it was called in the beginning. The word *rational* means different things to different people. For instance, some people believe that the word rational means something too intellectual, cold and unemotional. Some other people think that rational means against God and religion. More confusion is created because some people even went to the extent of believing that rational therapy was a form of classical rationalism in philosophy. In philosophy, rationalism is the doctrine which holds that reason or intellect, rather than the senses, is the real source of knowledge. Therefore, a rationalist in philosophy is one who believes that reason is the prime and absolute criterion of deciding what is true and *should* be the goal of life.

As Ellis never intended to suggest even remotely any of these meanings of the word 'rational' when he originally called his system of psychotherapy 'rational therapy'; he subsequently regretted the choice of his word. Anyway, when he used the word 'rational' to describe his system of psychotherapy, he went by the meaning of the word rational given in the dictionary: 'of, based, on, or derived from reasoning; sensible; practical; judging soundly'.

However, of all the meanings people gave to the word 'rational', none is more detrimental to the spread of REBT than the meaning: against God and religion. Many people who believe in God and religion doubt whether it is worthwhile to seek help of REBT. Their misgivings about REBT may reduce if they read Ellis' views on this topic in detail.

Atheism and REBT

A large part of Ellis' education was a result of what he taught himself by voraciously reading books throughout his student days. In keeping with this practice, at the age of 12, he happened to read a book on physical geography and became an atheist because he felt that he was cheated by religion and its account of creation. Further, he followed the footsteps of Bertrand Russell and liberated himself from all religious and supernatural beliefs.

His interest in philosophy and scientific outlook taught him that it is not possible to prove or disprove the existence of God and the supernatural. Consequently, a die-hard atheist is also open to the charge of unscientific thinking and dogmatism. As Ellis was against unscientific thinking and any kind of dogmatic and absolutistic thinking, he could take the agnostic stand which states that it is impossible to know whether God and the supernatural exists or not. However, he did not subscribe to this stand because he believed that although the existence of God and the supernatural cannot be disproved, the probability that their existence can be proved is so low (i.e., 0.0000001 per cent) that it is quite scientific to say that he was a probabilistic atheist.

His main charge against religion was that it involves a belief in and dependence on some supernatural power whose existence has never been proved. Man's dependence on any such supernatural power is incompatible with all the goals of mental health promulgated by psychotherapists.

Religious and supernatural beliefs are absolutistic, dogmatic and antiscientific. According to REBT, emotional disturbance is also caused by absolutistic, dogmatic and unscientific musturbatory ideologies. The sovereign remedy for emotionally disturbed people is to teach them to surrender dogmatic and unscientific beliefs in God and the supernatural. Once they are liberated from such beliefs, it will not be very difficult to help them get rid of their absolutistic musturbatory ideologies and achieve emotional stability. Ellis was so convinced about this remedy for emotional disturbance that he even wrote an article, 'Atheism: A Cure for Neurosis' (Ellis, 1978), to propagate his views on this subject.

Pastoral Counselling and REBT

It is understandable if religious people have serious reservations about the use of REBT in the resolution of their emotional problems. Richard L. Wessler (1984), who was at one time a follower of Ellis and an outstanding practitioner of REBT, wrote an article to argue that pure REBT was inappropriate for pastoral counselling. According to him, neither Ellis, the therapist, nor the whole of REBT is compatible with pastoral counselling. However, he admits that certain parts of REBT are compatible with pastoral counselling and one can bridge the gap between psychotherapy and religion by focusing on those parts. He also suggests that cognitive appraisal therapy (CAT), a system of psychotherapy invented by him that offers a modified version of REBT, can be used in pastoral counselling. Of course, Ellis (1984) wrote another article and rebutted Wessler's arguments one by one. We need not go into the details of his rebuttal. Suffice it to say, rebellious Ellis evoked a considerable opposition from laymen and learned psychotherapists as well.

One probable cause of religious people's opposition to REBT can be traced to another article by Ellis (1971), 'The Case Against Religion: A Psychotherapist's View'. In this article, at the very outset, Ellis stated that it is not correct to say that religion means a philosophy of life or a code of ethics. Even an atheist has some kind of philosophy and some code of ethics. Many atheists have more rigorous philosophies and moral principles than most believers of God and religion. Hence, religion implies man's dependence on some supernatural power.

As a psychotherapist, Ellis found man's dependence on any supernatural power detrimental to his mental health. Broadly speaking, the concept of mental health includes many traits and behaviours such as self-interest, social interest, tolerance, acceptance of ambiguity, acceptance of reality, commitment, risk-taking, self-acceptance, rationality and scientific thinking. Surely, not all mentally healthy people have all the mentioned traits. People who are seriously deficient in these traits are to be regarded as mentally disturbed. Most of the people who believe in some supernatural power usually depend on that power and adopt the views preached by the recognized advocates of that power. As a result, they fail to develop their own views independently. This is more likely to happen if they are followers of a strongly organized religion. Such people find it difficult to cultivate the traits which characterize good mental health.

In essence, Ellis' thesis was based on the idea that a religious man by faithfully adopting the 'right' views preached by his religion becomes rigid, bigoted and dogmatic. It is the inflexibility of his thinking that makes him susceptible to emotional disturbance. There is nothing new or very shocking about this thesis, as it is expressed by many critics of religion. For example, in many of his writings Bertrand Russell (1930, 1946) has emphasized the idea that religion has, on balance, done more harm than good to human beings by seeking to suppress the spirit of free inquiry and frank criticism.

A.C. Grayling (2004), an outstanding British philosopher, states his objection to religion very neatly in his book, *What Is Good*? He says,

> In every case fundamentalists, whether or not they use the gun and the bomb in defence or furtherance of their views, are opposed to democracy, liberal pluralism, multiculturalism, religious toleration, secularism, free speech and equal rights for women. They reject the discoveries of modern science in the fields of physics and biology, and assert the literal and universal truth of their ancient holy writings. (pp. 92–93)

Indeed, one wonders whether this excerpt is from A.C. Grayling's writing or by Ellis. All that Ellis did in presenting his case against religion is to explain elaborately how the dogmatic thinking of devoutly religious people is vulnerable to emotional disturbance. By doing so, he opened a Pandora's Box and his critics took him to task for his blasphemy.

Religiosity, Not the Religion

What was Ellis' contention? Did he really think that being religious meant being irrational and emotionally disturbed? Certainly not! As a psychotherapist, he believed that not all religious people are emotionally disturbed. Rather, it is devout religiosity that tends to be harmful to man's emotional health. By devout religiosity, Ellis meant a pietistic, rigid and dogmatic belief in and reliance upon some kind of supernatural, divine or 'higher' power. It also means strict obedience to and fanatical worship of that hypothesized power. This kind of absolutistic religiosity creates emotional disturbance which is usually a result of rigid, absolutistic musturbatory thinking.

To make this view more explicit, he revised his earlier article and published it under the title 'The Case Against Religiosity' (Ellis, 1983). The revision was partly prompted by his realization that he took a very dim view of the mental health of religionists. Ellis admitted that sometimes religion is defined as a philosophy of life involving an ethical code. This vague, general or mild definition of religion is probably a natural part of the human condition and is very unlikely to be related to man's mental health. However, if religion means a way of life, it would be difficult to say who can be called a thoroughly non-religious person! Anyway, Ellis was opposed to religiosity—devout and dogmatic belief in a theological or even atheistic creed. Besides, he no longer believed that religion creates emotional disturbance.

Secular dogmatism: Significantly enough, Ellis went one step ahead and suggested that just as religion can be dogmatic, even communism, fascism, closed-minded capitalism or any other 'ism' can inculcate a mentality among its devout followers which is antithetical to good mental health. Even pious adherents of a secular cause, who don't believe in any supernatural power, can become emotionally disturbed if they cling to some absolutistic rules of conduct and hate themselves when they fail to follow those rules. They may also hate others who don't follow those rigid rules. This intolerance of oneself and others creates unhealthy emotions such as extreme anxiety, depression, self-hatred and rage. Thus, Ellis' main thesis was that rigid and dogmatic beliefs—religious or secular—endanger our mental or emotional health. The new title itself underlines the idea that mental health is likely to be endangered by blind devotion to any dogmatic ideology.

Objectivism: According to Ellis, even those who devoutly believe in Marxism, psychoanalysis or any other secular creed may dogmatically insist that some political, economic, social or philosophic view offers answers to all the important questions and, therefore, *must* be adopted by all human beings who want to lead a good life. An example will make this idea clear. Ayn Rand, well-known novelist and philosopher, was an atheist. Ellis believed that her philosophy called Objectivism was unrealistic, rigid and dogmatic. He wrote the book, *Is Objectivism a Religion?* (Ellis, 1968), which critically examines her philosophy. The point to note is that as Objectivism is extremist and dogmatic, Ellis considered it a religion! He went to the extent of saying that if he piously and rigidly believes in REBT, then he is afflicted with religiosity as well!

To summarize, Ellis' hypothesis was that a belief in any rigid, inflexible and dogmatic cause or cult is likely to affect the mental health of man adversely. When he asserted that atheism is a cure for neurosis, he hypothesized that unbelief and scepticism promote mental health.

REBT and Religions

Although REBT philosophy and religious philosophy are considered separate domains, the theoretical underpinnings of certain concepts of REBT are related to religious ideologies too.

REBT and Christianity: Ellis' position vis-à-vis religion did not suggest that REBT is against religion and therefore religious people cannot be benefited by it. As he made a distinction between religion and religiosity, religious people can and do find REBT useful in overcoming their emotional disturbance. That is why many Christian counsellors such as John Powell, Bred Johnson and Stevan Nielson practise REBT quite effectively. Counsellors such as Paul Hauck, Hank Robb, Raymond DiGiuseppe and Howard Young have helped religious persons by offering them 'rational' ideas in Christian terms.

There is nothing surprising in the fact that REBT is in agreement with some parts of Christian philosophy. Ellis had created REBT by borrowing some of the main ideas, such as, USA, from a famous Christian theologian Paul Tillich. Besides, REBT incorporates many ideas taken from divergent teachings of Gautam Buddha (an ascetic), Epicurus (a hedonist), Epictetus (a pagan stoic), Marcus Aurelius (a persecutor of Christians), Brauch Spinoza (a pantheist), Bertrand Russell (an atheist) and several others.

In his article, 'Can Counseling Be Christian?', Ellis (1997) pointed out that as many religiously oriented counsellors have shown, REBT can certainly be done in a Christian manner. Some of the rational philosophies taught in REBT are also preached by the New Testament and other Christian writings. For instance, REBT's philosophy of USA, unconditional other acceptance (UOA), HFT, wanting but not needing the approval and love of others, and accepting oneself with one's own emotional disturbance have Christian counterparts.

REBT and Judaism: Does it mean that the basic tenets of REBT are in harmony with some of the teachings of only one religion, namely, Christianity? Certainly not! Ronald Pies (2000), a clinical professor of psychiatry, in his article, 'Symptoms, Suffering and Psychodynamics: A Personal Journey from REBT to the Talmud', recalls that his Jewish mother, a psychiatric social worker, introduced him to REBT in his early teens. Subsequently, he studied REBT to find out its link with Jewish philosophy. He then realized that in many aspects, Ellis' cognitive approach was similar to the views expressed in Talmudic Judaism. He especially underlines the fact that the Talmud urges a man not to judge himself as a wicked person. How similar is it to Ellis' concept of acknowledging and even condemning one's bad behaviour but not judging and labelling one's totality or oneself! Further, Ronald Pies declares that the cognitive approach is truly the deepest and most radical therapy that one can bring to bear upon a psychiatric symptom.

REBT and Buddhism: Let it not be construed that Christianity and Judaism are the only religions that contain many of the basic philosophical tenets of REBT. If one takes the trouble of carefully studying the scriptures of almost all the major religions of the world such as Hinduism, Buddhism, Islam, etc., one would come across many parallels between their teachings and some fundamental principles of REBT. Ellis agreed that there are unusual similarities between his views and His Holiness the Dalai Lama's views expressed in his book, *The Art of Happiness* (His Holiness the

Dalai Lama, & Cutler, 1998). In fact, there are 20 techniques of reducing emotional disturbance and achieving happiness which are endorsed by both Ellis and the Dalai Lama. For example, both believe that unconditional acceptance of self and others lead to less fear, more openness and honesty and more authentic relationships.

Yet, another example of how REBT can be blended with religious beliefs is provided in the article, 'The Interface Between Rational Emotive Behaviour Therapy (REBT) and Zen', authored by Kwee and Ellis (1998). It describes how REBT agrees with several aspects of Zen Buddhism. Especially, it shows how the narrative techniques of Zen by means of *Koans* (e.g., analogies, metaphors, parables) and REBT's cognitive, emotive and behavioural methods are, to some extent, complementary to each other. Hence, Zen techniques, when separated from their mystical and utopian aspects, can be included in the practice of REBT.

REBT and Hinduism: Like Christianity, Judaism and Buddhism, attempts have been made to explicate the links between REBT premises and the doctrines of Hindu scriptures. In the book *Counselling and Psychotherapy with Religious Persons: A REBT Approach* (Nielsen, Johnson, & Ellis, 2001), Ellis has mentioned that some elements of Hindu religious traditions and practices are congruent with REBT theory and practice. As REBT emphasizes on an extensive amount of teaching and education, it shows resemblance to the teachings and practices of many religions. Ellis supported his view by mentioning the quotes of religious scriptures that endorse teaching as a religious enterprise. He quotes, from the Rig Veda (Hindu), 'One not knowing a land asks for one who knows it, he goes forward instructed by the knowing one. Such, indeed, is the blessing of instruction, one finds a path that leads him straight onward' (Rig Veda 10.32.7, p. 25).

The Bhagavad Gita and REBT: The Bhagavad Gita, the very influential spiritual Hindu scripture, has been widely studied by both Eastern and Western scholars in the contexts of philosophy, theology, literature and psychology.

Ellis' views: Ellis accepted that Indian philosophy contained a good deal of overlap with REBT, but he was of a view that Eastern thinkers very frequently carry their own ideas to unrealistic extremes (Phadke, 1968–2003). His main objection was to the term *Nishkam Karma*, which is the ideal path to realize the truth. It advocates selfless or desireless action and encourages the person to perform the action without any expectation or desire of fruits or results.

REBT makes a distinction between expectation (desire) and demand. On contrary to *Nishkam Karma*, it encourages the person to keep expectations or desires while doing our work. However, it cautions the person from turning expectations (desires) into demands since absolutistic demands lead to emotional disturbance. Ellis has mentioned this view explicitly in a book called *A New Guide to Rational Living* (Ellis & Harper, 1975). He writes,

> According to the Hindu Classic the Bhagavad Gita, the strongest individual "has indifference to honor and insult, heat and cold, pleasure and pain. He feels free from attachment." A few select individuals may find this worthy ideal. But we doubt whether many humans could ever attain it. To lean so far over backwards to get rid of psychological pain that you also eradicate all pleasure does not seem too rational to us. By all means, try, if you will, to eliminate your extreme, unrealistic, self-defeating desire; but not desire itself! (p. 95)

Ellis also noted his opinion in his correspondence with Phadke (1968–2003) when the thinkers talk about abandoning attachments, instead of, as REBT says, 'abandoning need'. REBT encourages people to have strong desires but not dire needs.

It is significant to note that Dr David Burns (1985), a well-known contributor to cognitive behaviour therapy (CBT) is more explicit in giving credit to Eastern philosophy. He mentioned that it is in fact the 'need' for love that often deprives the person of the intimacy he most desires. Burns drew this insight from Eastern philosophy, which suggests that you can't really gain what you want until you give up the idea that you 'need' it. Unlike Burns, Ellis never gave credit of the concept 'wanting but not needing' explicitly to Eastern philosophy. In his talks and workshops, he mentioned it but his focus was on to point out (Phadke, 1968–2003) that Eastern philosophers usually take things to great extremes and consequently throw out the baby with the bathwater.

Different Interpretations

Phadke (1968–2003) had attempted to study the discourses of Bhagavad Gita in detail. He referred to the second chapter of Bhagavad Gita which says,

> Do the work by abandoning attachments and with an even mind in success and failure, for evenness of mind is called Yoga.

His suggestion to Ellis was to substitute the word 'need' in place of the word attachment. In that case, the advice becomes the anti-musturbatory philosophy of REBT. But, Ellis viewed the attachment and non-attachments as 'either/or' extremes and did not accept the interpretation. However, Ellis (1994) refined his insights on attachment more specifically in the second edition of the book, *Reason and Emotion in Psychotherapy*. In his view, 'either/or' extreme position creates emotional trouble as the person has to be unattached and uninvolved. Hence, Ellis tried to solve this problem with the and/also continuum. The person can be over-attached to his desires (demand or compulsive *musturbation*) or he can be totally non-attached to desires (desireless). Ellis proposed that the better option is to attach distinctly (involved) and non-attached (not desperately involved). Ellis noted that this position would be more self-actualizing.

Anasakti Yoga and REBT

Authors of this book feel that the concept of 'Anasakti Yoga' devised by Mohandas Karamchand Gandhi (Mahatma Gandhi) shows resemblance to the REBT philosophy. 'Anasakti Karma' is a philosophy advocated by Gandhi (1984) that essentially encourages non-attachment to the fruits of one's actions. Gandhi clarified that the principle of renunciation of the fruit of action does not mean indifference to fruits. He explained (1984) that 'Renunciation means absence of hankering after fruit, because attachment, worry, haste affect our nervous system and upset the balance of our mind' (p. 7). It is not unnatural to feel happy about the good outcome of one's hard work, but it is wasteful, both spiritually and psychologically, to invest one's emotions and energy in fretting over the results instead of focusing on perfecting the work. People who practise Anasakti Yoga are still completely engaged in and dedicated to their actions and work, but without any attachment to the outcome.

There are many parallels between REBT's doctrine of desire and demand and non-attachment proposed by Anasakti Yoga. Like REBT, it encourages keeping desires, with non-attachment (i.e., without keeping absolutistic demand). Anasakti Yoga mediates the 'either/or' extremes and goes well with the view expressed by Ellis.

REBT with Religious People

It will be a mistake to think that REBT and religious beliefs are at loggerheads. On the contrary, Ellis co-authored a book, *Counselling and Psychotherapy with Religious Persons*, with Steven L. Nielsen and W. Brad Johnson (2001), who are religious psychologists. The book describes how a client who firmly believes in the sacred beliefs of his religion can be helped to overcome his mental disturbance by using REBT. For example, it gives clear-cut methods of disputing the client's absolutistic evaluative thinking—revealed in his awfulizing, demanding or musturbating, intolerable frustration and condemning man's totality—by using techniques which are congruent with his religious beliefs.

In this book, Steven L. Nielsen gives a good example of how, as a counsellor, he helped Deborach, a client who was strongly committed to her religious beliefs.

Case 7.1

Case of Deborach

> Deborach had increased her weight by 20 pounds during the time she was away from her home on a religious mission. When she returned home, her mother made no secret of the fact that she hated her fatness and was ashamed of her. She also told Deborach that she liked Ruth, her slim sister. Deborach was angry at her mother and demanded that her mother be more fair and stop insisting that she reduce her weight. Deborach had two problems. First, her mother was unfair to her. Second, she was troubled by her own anger at her mother—a self-created unnecessary problem.

Analysis of Case 7.1: During a counselling session, Deborach frankly told the counsellor that his Socratic method of disputing her belief that her mother *must* treat her fairly was not yielding any good result. The counsellor then changed his strategy. As a devoutly religious person, Deborach knew that even Isaac and Jacob, who were patriarchs, behaved unjustly with their children. Hence, if God could permit the patriarchs to behave unjustly with their children, was there any sense in demanding that Deborach's mother, who was an imperfect human being, *should* not be unjust to her. As Deborach had a firm belief in patriarchs, she realized the absurdity of her demanding that her mother *should* behave justly with her when even the patriarchs could easily behave unfairly with their children. This realization helped her to reduce her anger at her mother. Of course, the book also outlines how emotive and behavioural techniques can also be adapted for counselling religious clients.

Ellis' revised view: Let's go back to Ellis' case against devout religiosity. In view of the research findings regarding religion and mental health, Ellis revised his views about religion and devout religiosity.

He admitted that religious attitudes—even if they are extreme and absolutistic—can sometimes bring about good mental health. Perhaps, the important thing from the point of view of mental health is not whether people hold religious or non-religious beliefs. Rather, the important thing is what kind of religious or non-religious beliefs they hold. A considerable amount of research has shown that people who view God as a warm, caring and lovable friend, and who see their religion as supportive, are more likely to have positive results than those who take an unfavourable view of their God and religion.

Maybe, more research was necessary before we could say anything about the subject of religion and mental health with a reasonable amount of confidence. Ellis preferred to retain his hypothesis that absolutism is highly related to emotional disturbance, whereas unbelief and scepticism promote mental health. Indeed, some research findings support the idea that religious inflexibility and rigidity are associated with emotional problems.

However, it is worth noting that in his article, 'The Advantages and Disadvantages of Self-Help Therapy Materials', Ellis (1993) unhesitatingly stated that the Judeo-Christian Bible is a self-help book that has probably helped many people make more extensive and intensive personality and behavioural changes than all professional therapists combined. While paying tribute to Ellis for his disarming open-mindedness, one is tempted to add that what he says about the Judeo-Christian Bible can also be said about the Bhagavad Gita, the Koran and some other sacred books.

Humanistic-Existential Approach

Ellis' atheism, his rational and scientific approach to causes of psychological disturbance and his hard-hitting and down-to-earth language often gave rise to an impression in the minds of some psychologists and lay people that REBT is too cold, impersonal and overly rational.

Notwithstanding these misconceptions, Ellis had always been an adherent of humanism. Of course, there are many varieties of humanism. What kind of humanism did Ellis adopt and incorporate in REBT? It would be easy to guess the answer to the question if one bears in mind that Ellis had been an atheist and interested in the philosophy of human happiness since his adolescence. No wonder he called himself a secular humanist.

As a logical corollary of this stand, REBT is concerned with enhancing the welfare and happiness of all human beings who inhabit this world.

Human beings are free to pursue happiness, although REBT encourages them to aim at their both short-term and long-term happiness. It is often necessary to sacrifice short-term happiness for the sake of long-term happiness. It is extremely sceptical of all sorts of supernatural entities and powers. It even believes that the mental health of people who devoutly believe in such entities and powers may be adversely affected.

Though it is correct to say that REBT endorses humanistic psychology, there is a hitch because again the term humanism has two meanings—psychological and ethical. Although those two meanings are to some extent overlapping, they are different too.

According to the psychological meaning, the term humanism implies the study of the individual as a whole (instead of the study of his separate traits or performances) with a view to helping him live a happy, meaningful, self-actualizing and creative life in this world. Roughly speaking, this is the meaning of the term humanism according to the Association for Humanistic Psychology and similar other organizations.

On the other hand, the ethical meaning of the term humanism refers to the formulation of guidelines for people to live their lives. Those guidelines emphasize human interest rather than the interest of some sort of a presumed natural order or God. This is the meaning of the term humanism endorsed by the American Humanistic Association and similar other organizations.

The humanism of REBT includes both these concepts. The common factor in these two concepts is that they accept that people are human and, as such, they are fallible and have limited powers. REBT asserts that no antisocial or obnoxious behaviour of any man makes him damnable or subhuman. Unfortunately, the psychological humanism advocated by the Association for Humanistic Psychology has not always adhered to scientific outlook and methods. At least some of its followers preach very anti-scientific things such as astrology, magic, extrasensory perception (ESP) and what not.

The ethical humanism advocated by the American Humanistic Association strictly adheres to scientific outlook and methods. REBT is more at home with this approach. Incidentally, it may be added that in 1971, the American Humanistic Association bestowed on Ellis, its Humanist of the Year Award.

However, just as REBT is humanistic, it is existentialist too. Like all kinds of existentialism, REBT sees every man as a holistic, goal-directed individual who is important in the world just because he is human; he is alive; and he is unique. REBT does not hesitate to place human beings in the centre of the universe and of their own emotional life.

As REBT is wedded to scientific outlook and methods, it rejects the idea that the universe and man's life have any inherent meaning. At the same time, it believes that man can give meaning and purpose to his life. Similarly, he can choose his goals and also choose to work for achieving those goals. Of course, he can also choose not to have any specific long-term goals and therefore not to choose to work to achieve such goals! The key concept here is that of choice. Indeed, human beings have, to a very large extent, freedom to choose their thoughts, feelings and actions. Of course, REBT does not claim that their freedom of choice in this respect is totally unrestricted. On the contrary, it does admit that some behaviour of human beings may be partly caused by biosocial and other factors.

Yet, human beings have ample freedom to unconditionally accept themselves, others and the conditions under which they live and then to create or construct their helping behaviour for their own well-being and happiness.

Sane Morality

Ellis allied himself with the broad objective of ethical humanism expounded by the American Humanistic Association and believes that humans had better give priority to protecting and fulfilling their interests over the interests of inanimate nature of lower animals or of some otherworldly powers. This view is not a license to human beings to be insensitive and cruel to animals. Nor does it mean a license to show disrespect to other people and their views or ideologies.

As human beings live in some or other society, they have to obey at least some essential moral rules. Indeed, Ellis did offer two main rules of morality. If they appear somewhat different from the traditional rules of morality, it is because they are proposed by a psychologist who was probably born and reared to be a rebellious.

Two Rules of Morality

First rule: Ellis's first rule of morality is that a man had better be true to his own self. Therefore, he recommends us first to *safeguard our self-interests, be kind to ourselves and love ourselves*. To safeguard one's own interests means to be realistic while dealing with others. However, it does not encourage us to be selfish. It is the only way to ensure that in this world, there is at least one person who is kind to you and looks after your own interest.

If a man always behaves kindly to others and helps others to achieve their objectives at his owns cost, what will be the likely outcome in most instances? As he lives in a society of humans and not of angels or Gods, most of the time he will be a loser! Although some people will reciprocate his kind and considerate behaviour befittingly, majority of people will take his kindness as weakness and exploit him in a shamelessly selfish manner. Then, not only will he hate those ungrateful people but will also hate himself for allowing them to exploit him. Considering this reality about the behaviour of humans in general, it is advisable first to safeguard your self-interest, be kind to yourself and love yourself.

Second rule: What would probably happen if human beings follow only the first of the two rules of morality set forth by Ellis? Obviously, they will create a dog-eat-dog society in which they themselves will not like to live in. Therefore, human beings had better follow the second rule of morality put forward by Ellis. There is nothing new about his second rule. It is called the golden rule and is preached by almost all the major religions in the world. It advises a man to do unto others as he would like them to do unto him. Here is Ellis' version of that ancient golden rule: '*Do not commit any deed that needlessly, definitely and deliberately harms others*'. In short, the rule enjoins a man not to behave with others in such a way that he would not want them behave with him.

Ellis insisted that people had better follow his first rule of morality but at the same time follow the second rule too. The practice of following both the rules will ensure that human beings first look after their own self-interests but not at the expense of their fellow citizens.

Sequences of the rules: You may wonder why not change the sequence of Ellis' two rules of morality? Why not first look after the interests of other people and then take care of one's own interests? One answer to this question is already given here. Namely, often a self-sacrificer is likely to be exploited by other people, and, as a result, he will be a loser. Then he may hate those who exploit him and finally hate himself too! Hence, it will be self-defeating to put the interest and happiness of others ahead of your own happiness and self-interest.

There is yet another answer to this question. It is founded on the principle that the only purpose of being good to others and helping them and refraining from harming them is that thereby you will increase the probability (though not create any certainty) that others too will be good and helpful to you and not harm you. This is a sane, secular, non-religious and non-spiritual way of looking at morality. It will work very well if you happen to live in the society of angels. Angels are probably the creatures who will be kind to you when you are kind to them. However, you happen to live in a society of human beings, and they are different creatures. Perhaps, some human beings will be kind to you and keep from harming you needlessly because you are kind to them and don't harm them needlessly. They may sacrifice themselves for you because you have done many good things to them even at the cost of your self-interest. Only some people will behave with you in such a grateful way.

On the contrary, you will realize that many people will not show you any gratitude. They will behave in an unkind, unfair and even exploitative manner with you. This is so because many human beings are stupid, ignorant and emotionally disturbed. Therefore, self-sacrifice had better not be made the first principle of morality. If you thoughtlessly practise self-*sacrificism*, you may wind up by defeating your own goals and interests.

It is unrealistic to presume that when you sacrifice your goals and interests for the sake of others, they will always sacrifice their self-interest and goals for your requirements when you are in difficult situations. In a human society, your self-sacrifice tends to encourage others to develop dependence on you. In addition, when you realize that other people don't return your kindness, you are likely to hate yourself for being weak and also hate those who behave ungratefully, unkindly and even unjustly with you.

In view of the selfish, unkind and exploitative nature of the vast majority of human beings, it is sensible to give priority to your happiness and self-interest. Even the second principle of morality does not absolutely forbid you from harming others because in our competitive world, it is almost impossible to achieve your goals without harming others to some extent. Therefore, the second principle of morality urges you to be kind to others and not do any harm to them needlessly, definitely and deliberately, unless you don't mind being a loser in life!

Of course, it is possible that you do a lot of sacrifices for safeguarding the interest, welfare and growth of people you care and love. Sometimes you may like to be good to some people even at the cost of your self-interest just because you love them. That is your choice. However, when you behave in this way, no question of morality is involved. If you are kind to a man and help him because you love him, you may be a loving person, but this choice of yours does not make you a moral or immoral person. In such situations, you enjoy your self-sacrificing activities and expect nothing in return from those you care and love.

Perhaps, Ellis' two rules of morality or at least their sequence are at variance with customary and religious concepts of morality. They are even contrary to the view of Alfred Adler who placed social interest above self-interest. However, it may be interesting to learn that Heinz Ansbacher, a leading practitioner of Alfred Adler's individual psychology, told Ellis through personal communication (Phadke, 1968–2003) that in practice, Alfred Adler and his clients normally put self-interest first and social interest a closer second.

Man's Worth

Russell's view: In his celebrated book, *The Conquest of Happiness*, Bertrand Russell (1930) makes some very perceptive comments on the universally acclaimed virtue of modesty. According to him, it is questionable whether excessive modesty is beneficial or harmful. Usually, a modest man is afraid to undertake even those tasks that he is quite capable of performing well. He requires a great deal of encouragement to try to do things that are not very difficult. He feels that others are better than him, and hence they will surpass him in many respects. Consequently, he envies other people, feels ill towards them and makes himself unhappy.

In view of these disadvantages of excessive modesty, Bertrand Russell recommends that it is wise to rear a man to believe that he is a fine fellow. No psychotherapist can deny that Bertrand Russell's warning about the disadvantage of too much modesty is well founded. All present-day psychotherapies concur with the view that a man's evaluation of his own worth plays a very crucial role in his individual and social life. If he holds an extremely poor opinion of his own worth, he will belittle himself, and this will adversely affect his day-to-day functioning and make him feel all the more miserable.

Before getting trained as a psychoanalyst, Ellis was practising as a marriage and family counsellor. Since then, he had observed how a man's self-respect plays an important role even in his love and sex problems. That is why in an article, 'Unhealthy Love: Its Causes and Treatment', Ellis (1973) he wrote that the main problem of love is how much does a man accept and respect himself and how much does he care for his partner.

Even the basic issue underneath the human sex problem is to what extent a man considers himself worthwhile or worthless.

No wonder then, almost all psychotherapists use a variety of methods to help a man develop self-respect. Some other names for the concept of 'self-respect' are 'ego-strength', 'self-confidence', 'positive self-image', 'self-esteem', 'personal worth' and 'sense of identity'. The goal of psychotherapists who encourage man to develop a good deal of respect for himself is to help him evaluate his worth or value himself positively. That is exactly what Bertrand Russell means when he says that it is better to raise a man to believe that he is a fine fellow.

Self-respect: How does one help a man develop self-respect? One method of achieving this objective is to help a man concentrate on his good traits and his noteworthy performance in some tasks. For instance, if a student devalues himself and considers worthless because his performance in the academic sphere is just average or even below average compared to his friends, one can help him focus on his sincerity, loyalty and eagerness to help others when they are in difficulty. In addition, one can help him concentrate on his excellent achievements in some sport, hobby, etc. Yet another method is to encourage him to be an outstanding achiever in some tasks or worthy pursuits. Again, the basic idea behind this approach is that if a man proves that he is very successful in some walk of life, he will evaluate himself positively and consider himself a worthwhile person. Once he begins to think that he is a worthwhile human being, he will have fewer difficulties in socializing with others. As he becomes more and more successful in social life, his sense of being a worthwhile person will be reinforced.

Ayn Rand's view: As an outstanding example of this approach to build a man's self-respect, one can mention Ayn Rand's philosophy of objectivism (Rand & Branden, 1964). According to this philosophy, a man can create and maintain his self-esteem only by cultivating two traits. First, in order to deserve the right to live and be happy, a man *must* develop a belief that he is competent to live. Second, he can acquire and sustain the belief that he is quite competent to live by remaining busy in the process of growth as well as in the process of increasing his efficacy. At this point, it is necessary to underline the idea that continuously being involved in the process of one's own growth and also in the process of increasing one's own competence are not merely desirable activities, but they are absolutely necessary activities for building and maintaining one's self-esteem.

Will this and similar other methods help a man boost up his ego-strength and make him believe that he is a worthwhile person? Yes, often they will. Will a man's self-respect founded on good traits, success and achievements help him reduce his emotional vulnerability and improve his efficacy and happiness? Most probably, it will.

Ellis and Branden: For many years, Ellis wrongly thought that Nathaniel Branden, once a leading exponent of Ayn Rand's objectivism, was a follower of the self-esteem school of thought, so to speak. This means that Ellis thought that Nathaniel Branden also believed that people liked themselves when they are achievers. However, after corresponding with him, Ellis realized his own mistake. As a matter of fact, Nathaniel Branden urges people to select and accomplish goals in a responsible way. A responsible way of accomplishing something means to work for goals and values having good character and social responsibility.

Ellis thought that Nathaniel Branden's view (Branden, 1970) is a somewhat better version of the self-esteem school of thought. Still, Ellis did not think it is advisable to make accomplishments of even responsibly chosen targets, a prerequisite for accepting oneself. The reason was that the essence of various approaches to building a man's self-worth (the approaches which we have lumped together under the title 'self-respect school of thought', though there is no such distinctly labelled school of thought) is to help a man believe that he has a value or worth because he behaves intelligently, correctly and competently. But any attempt to judge a man's totality, his being or his very existence and to call him a worthy or worthless person on the basis of his good or bad possessions or performance is beset with many difficulties.

Difficulties in judging totality: Ellis had mentioned various reasons for why not to judge the totality of the person. Some of them are mentioned here.

1. Evaluating a man's totality or worth by rating the various traits of his personality is like trying to construct a building on a very shaky foundation. The very traits that are rated do not remain constant; they are subject to change throughout a man's lifetime. How can such changing process be correctly measured?

2. To evaluate a characteristic or trait as good or bad is to neglect the fact that there is no absolute standard to judge any trait. The utility of a trait varies from time to time and from culture to culture.

3. In order to evaluate a man's worth, it is necessary to judge his every good and bad act. It is not possible to do so. Suppose a man helps a blind person cross the road also tries to rescue about a hundred people from a building which is on fire. How does one rate these

two acts of that man? Similarly, a man tells a lie to his boss and also tells a lie to his wife. Can these two acts be accurately rated? How much additional information will be required to judge that these two acts are indeed bad?

4. How can we quantify a man's various good and bad acts? Is it possible to add up his score on various bad acts and then finally to determine his score showing his final worth? It is not really justifiable to arrive at any such final score when the goodness or badness of at least some traits is debatable.

5. Is it possible to find out all the characteristics of a man and then to evaluate them? Very unlikely! Hence, any evaluation of a man's totality is bound to be partial and hence defective.

6. If a man gets a very poor total rating, what does it imply? Does it mean that he is born a worthless person, will remain so forever and therefore deserves to be punished? These implications are likely to be harmful than helpful.

7. If a man is considered 'good' because he has good traits, what does it really mean? It means that he is good because he has those traits that are defined as good in a certain society. This is an arbitrary method of considering certain traits good and then regarding a man 'good' because he has arbitrarily defined good traits. When his total personality is labelled as good, even his arbitrarily defined good traits begin to appear more good or valuable (than they really may be) to the members of the society which has defined those traits as good in the first place.

   Similarly, if a man is considered 'bad' only because he has bad traits, what does it really mean? It means he is bad only because he has traits that are defined as bad by members of a certain society. Again, this is obviously an arbitrary method of evaluating certain traits as bad and then regarding a man 'bad' because he has those so-called bad traits. In this way, once a man's whole personality is branded as a bad man, even his arbitrarily defined bad traits begin to appear worse or of no value to the members of the society which has originally defined those traits as bad. Naturally, those people may consider that man worse than he may be. The problem with labelling a man as a 'good man' or as a 'bad man' is that there is no way to define either the goodness or badness of a man's totality.

8. There is another method of rating a man's total personality. This method does not judge a man on the basis of his good or bad traits at all. It evaluates a man on the basis of his sheer aliveness.

According to this method, a man is good or worthwhile just because he is human and alive. There is another version of this method. According to this version, a man is good or worthwhile just because he is a human being and some God or deity in whom he believes, accepts, loves and grants grace to all human beings. This method may be found useful by some people for considering themselves good and worthwhile. The problem with this method is that it regards all human beings as good and worthwhile without leaving scope for considering any body bad. Moreover, this method is not useful for non-believers. Anyway, these two methods of rating a man's essence or totality appear to be palliative rather than curative.

9. Perhaps, our faulty use of language creates the problem of finding out a way to evaluate a man's total personality. Semanticists often point out that just as two pens are not identical, nor two individuals are similar. Therefore, any generalized statement about pens or individuals is bound to be inaccurate. Of course, on the basis of some factual evidence, we may correctly say that your brother possess some outstanding talents. But to say that your brother is an outstandingly talented man is an overgeneralized and hence incorrect statement.

Although, it may be inevitable to make some general statements about objects and human beings, it is advisable to bear in mind that we can fairly know and talk about specific characteristics of objects and people. However, when we make a global statement about a man, we commit the mistake of overgeneralization.

10. Suppose there are many mangoes, bananas and oranges in one basket. How can we add and divide mangoes, bananas and oranges and find out a single general rating of that basket of fruit? Similarly, as human traits are different, how can we really add and divide different traits of a man and then give a single general rating of that man?

Let us agree that it is not possible to evaluate a man's totality, his being or his very existence on the basis of his good or bad performance. Suppose psychologists really invent a method of evaluating a man's totality which overcomes all these mentioned difficulties. Then will psychotherapists be able to help their clients to respect themselves and get rid of their self-doubts and anxiety?

It is not easy to answer this question affirmatively. The real problem with a global assessment of a man's worth is that such an assessment tends to make him feel insecure. Suppose a man's performance is adequately assessed and he is considered a good man on the basis of that assessment, he will still not be free from mental uneasiness. As he is considered a good man on the basis of his good performance, he may feel anxious about maintaining his good performance in the future and thereby proving that he is a good man at all times and under all circumstances. This anxiety may even affect his relations with himself and others.

On the other hand, suppose a man is considered a bad man on the basis of his bad performance, it will be difficult for him to be at peace with himself and with others too. He is likely to feel guilty and depressed about his being labelled a bad man and consequently he is also likely to perform poorly compared to his capabilities. This may even induce him to conclude wrongly that he really is a bad man.

In sum, if a man is judged either good or bad on the basis of his performance, he cannot be freed from mental distress.

Unconditional Acceptance

Unconditional Self-Acceptance (USA)

What then can be the solution to the emotional problem created by any attempt to assess and develop a man's self-respect, ego-strength, self-confidence, personal worth or sense of identity? A very elegant solution is put forth by Ellis. The fundamental premise of his approach to this tricky problem of a man's worth is that the very question posed by most of the modern psychotherapists is faulty. They think that if a man's self-acceptance appears to depend on his reasonably good performance in life and on maintaining good relations with people around him, how can he be helped to achieve these two goals?

We have seen that this approach does not solve a man's problem of self-acceptance. Therefore, Ellis put the problem before psychotherapists in this way: If a man's view of his own worth importantly affects his thoughts, feelings and activities, how to help him constantly evaluate himself so that in spite of his changeable good and bad performance and his good and bad relations with other people, he always accepts or respects himself?

Let us see how Ellis gradually evolved his answer to this question. Of course, he was in agreement with the renowned semanticist Alfred Korzybski's view that to label a man as 'good' or 'bad' is to commit the fallacy of overgeneralization. Ellis found a way by following the approach of existential philosophers. This approach was not new to him because his own analyst and psychoanalytical supervisor, Charles Hulbeck, had urged him to use existential philosophy in analysing and treating clients.

Subsequently, Ellis also got acquainted with the existential outlook of Paul Tillich and other eminent existential philosophers such as Martin Heidegger and Jean Paul Sartre. Consequently, he was convinced that the logical solution to the problem of man's worth was to abandon the method of rating a man's worth on the basis of his performance, and then to help him value himself on the basis of his very being or his existence.

Sometime in 1960, Ellis came across the writings of Robert S. Hartman (1959), who was a professor of philosophy and a business consultant. He had put forward excellent arguments against the idea of rating a man's totality. Ellis established a friendly link with him. Although Robert S. Hartman was living and teaching in Mexico, he visited Ellis in New York City for discussing topics of their common interest.

When Ellis began to adopt what could rightly be called Tillich–Hartman approach to the problem of man's worth, his main emphasis was on teaching a client that he was good because he was alive, was human and a unique individual. A man does not have to fulfil any condition such as being successful and competent or/and developing and maintaining good relations with other people, etc. In short, a client was encouraged and taught to unconditionally consider and accept himself as a good man.

Analysis of Case 5.1 in Light of USA

Teaching USA to Aditi: It is easy to understand how Ellis, who follows the footsteps of Tillich, Hartman and many other existentialists, will teach Aditi to inculcate the belief that even if she fails in her job interview and therefore does not get a job she has applied for, or for that matter any job, she can consider herself a 'good' person. Although, she may justifiably conclude that her performance in the interview was not satisfactory, her getting or not getting a job may reveal something about her extrinsic worth, that is, her worth in the practical world. However, this has nothing to do with her intrinsic worth. She will always be good because she is a human being, alive and is unique. In other words, her therapist will teach her to accept herself as a good person unconditionally, irrespective of her good or bad performances throughout life.

Logical difficulty: Usually Ellis found this method of restoring his client's worth quite useful, although occasionally he encountered a major difficulty. Some of his clients challenged the idea that a man is good and worthwhile just because he is a human being, alive and unique. How one can prove this belief? If somebody asserts that a man is bad or neutral (neither good nor bad) just because he is a living human being and is unique too, how can one logically refute this assertion? Indeed, if Aditi launches this kind of counter-attack on Ellis' arguments, how will he defend his existentialist stand?

Of course, Ellis can refute her idea that if she fails to do well in the interview, she will have to consider herself a bad or worthless person. However, this belief of Aditi cannot be logically proved. Nevertheless, what proof can Ellis offer to substantiate the belief that she is always intrinsically worthwhile to herself just because she is a living human being and she is unique?

Ellis' elegant solution: As Ellis continued to grapple with this problem, he thoroughly examined the very concept of man's worth. He came to the conclusion that the very question, 'What am I worth?' or 'How do I prove that I am a good person?' is a meaningless question!

Surely, one can give a sensible answer to the questions such as, 'What do you do?' 'What are your traits?' 'What is the value of your today's performance in the final badminton match?' These questions ask something about traits, characteristics or performance that can be observed and can be measured or rated. For example, answers to these questions may be like, 'I am a college student'; 'I possess good communication skills'; and 'My performance in the final badminton match today was excellent as I won it'. If anybody asks you, 'What is your worth or value?' how can you give any sensible answer to such a vague and indefinable question?

Therefore, Ellis arrived at the conclusion that it is preferable to solve the problem of human worth by giving up the idea of rating a man's worth. Accept the fact that you exist, and you are nothing but you! No doubt, you have many traits, and you can and had better rate them for practical purposes. For instance, your ability to walk, swim, dance, climb, etc. can be usefully evaluated. You may even present a profile of your personality in terms of your measurable or rateable traits. But don't forget that they are your traits still. Hence, refrain from concluding that because your traits are good and useful in practical life, you are good or worthwhile. Similarly, refrain from concluding that because your traits are bad and somewhat harmful in practical life, you are bad or worthless. This non-judgmental approach towards yourself will help you to feel relaxed and comfortable. At last, you are ready to ask yourself, 'What do I really want in my life? How do I go about getting what I want and avoiding what I don't want in my life?'

Thus, Ellis' main answer to the problem of man's worth is that it is a pseudo problem! Teach a man, says Ellis, to accept that he exists; his behaviour can be good or bad, but he or his totality, his being or his very existence cannot be good or bad. Does it mean that the concept of self-respect, self-confidence, ego-strength, etc., has no place in Ellis' view of man's worth? If a man plays badminton regularly and wins important matches, will it not increase his self-confidence?

Work-confidence: Ellis' answer to this question is that a man can increase his work-confidence or performance-confidence by rigorously practising a task. For example, a man who plays badminton regularly and wins important matches may develop a good deal of confidence that in the future he will continue to play well and win matches. The term work-confidence or performance-confidence aptly describes what a man can acquire or lose vis-à-vis any work or task. As any work or performance-confidence is based on experiences, it is at least to some extent undependable or shaky. The fact that a man has played badminton very well in the past does not guarantee that he will always play that game very well in the future. There could be so many reasons why he may fail to play that game well in the future. As a result, his confidence in his ability to play badminton successfully in the future is liable to go up and down. Even if he feels self-confident and accepts himself as a worthwhile person today because he plays badminton very well, he is still prone to feeling anxious and depressed about his performance in the future. His confidence in this aspect depends upon his ability to play badminton very well. As his confidence depends on something outside himself, namely, his good or bad performance, which can be called conditional self-confidence or conditional self-acceptance (CSA).

Self-acceptance: In view of this predicament, Ellis distinguished between work-confidence and self-confidence. According to him, self-confidence means a man's steady confidence in himself as a person, no matter whether he is able to do well at certain tasks. To make this concept more explicit, he preferred to use the term 'self-acceptance' instead of the term 'self-confidence'. To restate his concept precisely, self-acceptance means fully or completely accepting oneself without laying down any condition whatsoever for accepting oneself, which is called USA.

Now let us go back to the problem that Ellis may encounter while helping Aditi understand that she is always intrinsically worthwhile to herself just because she is a living human being and is unique. He can easily show her that even if she fails to do well in the job interview, she does not have to consider herself a bad or worthless person because this conclusion cannot be logically substantiated. By following the same line of argument, if she asserts that a human being is bad or neutral (neither good nor bad) just because he is a living human being and is unique too, how can Ellis refute her assertion? Indeed, he cannot logically disprove her assertion. If Ellis adopts the above elegant solution (mentioned before) to the problem of human worth, he will be able to free himself from the responsibility of proving that Aditi is always intrinsically worthwhile to herself. Ellis' solution drops the idea of rating a man's worth and focuses on rating only performances and acts of a man.

Accordingly, Ellis will agree that logically speaking, he can neither prove that she is worthwhile nor can he prove that she is worthless, as a man's worth cannot be rated or measured. All that she needs to do is to accept that she is a living human being and is unique. That is all! Then she can go on preparing for and giving more interviews, rating her performances in those interviews and learning to increase her performance or work-confidence until she gets a suitable job. Even if she fails to increase her work-confidence and fails to get a suitable job, she will not put herself down as a human being. Nor will she put herself on a pedestal as a great woman. On the contrary, she will always unconditionally accept herself and calmly go about increasing her work-confidence as and when necessary.

Two core concepts: Ellis' resolution of the problem of human worth involves two core concepts. First, it is impossible to rate a man's totality, his being or his very existence. Second, a man can continue to rate his performance as good or bad for practical purposes. It is true that even before Ellis developed his approach to the problem of man's worth, Carl Rogers was teaching his clients to attain self-acceptance or to develop unconditional positive regard for themselves. However, Ellis' concept of USA differs from Carl Rogers' concept of unconditional positive regard (Rogers, 1961).

Carl Rogers means to say that a man can accept himself just because he exists, and he can do so without referring to his achievements or any good behaviour. However, the term *unconditional positive regard* (which was, in fact, originally coined by him) is somewhat ambiguous. Usually, we respect or regard a man positively because of his good traits and achievements. Rogers' writings seem to mean or at least imply that a man can truly accept himself only when some other person, say a therapist, accepts him or loves him unconditionally. If so, then the Rogerian concept of unconditional positive regard seems to mean, at least partly, conditional positive regard. On the contrary, Ellis' concept of self-acceptance is completely free from the concept of conditional acceptance of oneself.

It is evident that Ellis' solution to the problem of man's worth surpasses even Hartman's existential stand. Hartman probably believed that a man has some intrinsic worth or value and that value can be measured. He even developed a test of human value. On the contrary, Ellis believed that the intrinsic worth or value of a man is unprovable. According to him, Hartman's test of a man's intrinsic value is not a valid assessment technique.

Ellis' work on USA: As Ellis was formulating and consolidating his ideas about man's intrinsic worth, he got an excellent opportunity to share them with some eminent scholars actively interested in axiology—a branch of philosophy dealing with values. Sometime in 1970, he was invited by Professor William Davis of the University of Tennessee at Knoxville to contribute a paper to the book, *Value and Valuation: Axiological Studies in Honour of Robert S. Hartman*, which was being edited by Professor Davis himself (1972). Ellis sized the opportunity and wrote the paper entitled, *Psychotherapy and the Value of a Human Being* (Ellis, 1972). Professor Davis was impressed by Ellis' paper and showed it to Hartman. When Hartman read the paper, he was so influenced by Ellis' innovative approach to the problem of man's worth that, as a professor of philosophy, he was ready to confer a PhD degree in philosophy on Ellis only on the basis of that paper. Of course, Ellis was extremely happy to know about the high praise Hartman had showered on him because philosophy was his hobby since the age of 16. Incidentally, Professor Davis' book was duly published by the University of Tennessee Press in 1972.

Indeed, Hartman had even invited Ellis to his home in Mexico with a view to continuing their debate. Unfortunately, Ellis could not go to Mexico before Hartman's demise. Nevertheless, Ellis still adheres to his views presented in this paper; however, over the years, he continued to add new arguments in favour of evaluating the performance and deeds of a man as against evaluating the totality or the very being of a man.

Elegant solution to Aditi: Granted that Ellis' resolution of the problem of man's intrinsic worth is thoroughgoing and logically sound, has not the usual practice of rating one's self-esteem or self-worth on the basis of one's performance and approval received from others some advantages also? What is wrong if Ellis encourages Aditi to visualize how proud and worthwhile she will feel by doing well in the interview, getting the job and being approved by others? Why not point out to her how her overall self-confidence or self-esteem will get a big boost if she secures the job? Why not show her that with increased self-esteem, she will be able to influence people and earn their approbation? These are just some ways in which Ellis can help her feel that she is a good and worthwhile human being. What is wrong with these and similar other methods of boosting a man's self-esteem?

It cannot be denied that if Ellis uses some of these methods of bolstering a man's ego-strength or self-confidence, she may be strongly motivated to give up her diffidence and anxiety and consequently she may do well in the interview. If she gets the job, she may feel great, do very well at her work and even become creatively involved in many other activities too. Moreover, it is normal and natural for a human being to rate his performance as well as his self, his totality or his being than to rate only his performance. One may even go further and say that if Ellis adopts some of the traditional methods to help her feel good about herself and also to feel that she is worthwhile, he can be complemented for aligning himself with a natural and normal human tendency.

If Ellis boosts Aditi's self-esteem and self-worth by showing her the advantages of doing well in the interview and getting the job, he faces a major risk. After all, nobody can assure Aditi that she will definitely succeed in the interview and get the job. In case she performs miserably in the interview and fails to secure the job, what will be her condition? As her self-esteem or self-worth is dependent on success, she is likely to think that she is worthless. She may also feel depressed, guilty and anxious. These unhealthy feelings will tend to confirm her belief that she is worthless.

Even if Aditi gets the job, her problem is only temporarily solved as she feels worthwhile only because of her achievement of getting the job. In order to feel worthwhile always and under all conditions, she has to be always successful in everything she will do in the future. Therefore, she will tend to develop the belief that she *must* be perfect in whatever she undertakes and gets the approval of others; or else, she is worthless. As a result, she may feel anxious most of the time. Her anxiety of failing and not being approved by significant people in her life will make her abnormally vigilant about her performance in all tasks. She will be always on her guard, so that she does not fail and prove that she is worthless. Unfortunately, the anxiety and tension created by her over watchfulness will interfere with and deteriorate her performance. In her desperate struggle to prove her worth by doing outstandingly well in all walks of life, she will sidetrack the main question: how can I live life happily? All this is because Ellis has helped her acquire only CSA). This means that she has learned to accept herself only to the extent that she is successful and capable of winning the appreciation of people she considers significant in her life.

On the contrary, if Ellis helps Aditi accept herself whether or not she is successful and whether she is appreciated or not, she will not feel excessively proud of her accomplishments or approval of others. Although she will certainly feel proud of her accomplishments and approval of others, she will not feel unhealthy emotions of depression, guilt and anxiety if she performs poorly at certain tasks and fails to win the appreciation of people she considers significant in her life. She will not take her performance in certain tasks as well as her failure to win the appreciation of significant people in her life. She will not condemn herself and wallow in the unhealthy emotions of self-loathing and self-pity.

Once she acquires this kind of USA, irrespective of her good and bad performances and also irrespective of other people's approval or disapproval, she will feel more at ease with herself and others as well. Besides, she will inculcate an attitude or philosophy that can be summarized as follows:

> If I succeed and earn the approval of others, I will have some advantages. Similarly, if I fail in some tasks and incur the disapproval of others, I will have some disadvantages. But success, approval, failure and disapproval reveal nothing about my intrinsic worth simply because there is no such thing as my intrinsic worth. I accept myself because I am human, alive and unique. Now how do I go about getting more of what I want and less of what I don't want.

Of course, it will not be easy for Aditi to learn only to rate her performance and deeds and not her totality or her being. Yet, she would be well advised to learn this difficult lesson so that it will help her become more happy and productive in the long run.

Unconditional Other Acceptance (UOA)

The central idea underlying Ellis' method of helping clients like Aditi is that although it is possible to rate a man's performance and traits, it is impossible to rate his overall personality, his totality or his being. This basic idea can have important implications for a man's relationships with other people too.

Analysis of Case 5.2 in Light of UOA

Teaching UOA to Vikram: Let us recall the main problem of our second case, Vikram. He feels intense anger with his boss because of his unfair ways of getting work done from his subordinates. By following Ellis' idea, Vikram can learn only to rate his boss' behaviour and may allow himself to feel annoyed (even strongly annoyed) at that unfair behaviour but, at the same time, to accept his boss because like all human beings, he is also fallible. Indeed, if Vikram learns to accept his boss unconditionally. Although he dislikes the boss' unfair behaviour, he will be able to focus on his main problem: how can I sanely communicate with my boss so that I can induce him to change his unfair methods of getting work done from me? If Vikram brings about this change in his attitude, it can be surmised that he has imbibed the philosophy of UOA. This philosophy will help Vikram accept his boss calmly irrespective of boss' bad behaviour—real or presumed!

Vikram will also reap a more generalized benefit by adopting the philosophy of UOA. He will find it easy to accept all other people unconditionally and deal with them in an unhostile manner, even when he dislikes some of their behaviour and traits.

On the contrary, Vikram's current philosophy about his boss' unfair behaviour is something like, 'I will accept my boss and consider him good if he is not unfair to me'. In short, Vikram's current philosophy can be called conditional other acceptance (COA). At present, this philosophy is making Vikram angry with his boss, who obviously is not behaving the way Vikram wants him to behave.

It is possible that Vikram learns to tackle his problem vis-à-vis his boss by adopting a philosophy which is different from the philosophy of COA. Vikram can adopt a somewhat over-optimistic (and hence quite unrealistic) philosophy that other people are 'good people' just because they are human, alive and unique. This philosophy may turn out to be helpful to him in practical life most of the time. However, it is not a commendable philosophy because it is unrealistic and unreliable. However, Ellis' philosophy of UOA is thoroughgoing and logical.

Unconditional Life Acceptance (ULA)

It is not at all surprising that the philosophy of USA and the philosophy of UOA are two of the most basic tenets of REBT. After all, REBT has its origins in the writings of some ancient and modern philosophers who have time and again pointed out that the acceptance of reality is the first step in overcoming any misfortune.

It is quite understandable if a man dislikes or even strongly dislikes some of his own or other people's behaviour. It is also not unreasonable if he abhors many conditions in the world. In fact, feeling frustrated about some aspects of himself, others and the world and life conditions can motivate him to change those aspects and live his life peacefully and happily. However, he will not be able to bring about the desirable changes in the undesirable aspects of the world if he does not accept those aspects unconditionally, without awfulizing about them and without creating unhealthy emotions in his mind in respect to those aspects.

Analysis of Case 5.3 in Light of ULA

Teaching ULA to Saniya: Now let us consider the main problem of our third case, Saniya. She is depressed because she believes that the task of consistently following the diet recommended by her doctor *must* not be too difficult instead, it *must* be very easy. As a result of this belief in her mind, she has made herself a victim of the philosophy of LFT. This philosophy, which is the source of discomfort disturbance, has made her extremely intolerant of the discomfort that can arise from the practice of consistently following her doctor's advice.

In other words, Saniya is not accepting the reality that if she wants to reduce her weight, she has to inculcate the philosophy of HFT so that she can consistently follow the diet prescribed by her doctor. Her current demand for ease and comfort can be countered by teaching her the philosophy of unconditional life acceptance (ULA). This is just another name for HFT.

If Saniya fully assimilates the philosophy of ULA, she will give up her demand for ease and comfort in the short run and consistently follow the diet prescribed by her doctor by focusing on the long-term goal of reducing her weight. Essentially, the philosophy of ULA allows a man to experience healthy emotions such as frustration, even as he willingly tolerates handicaps and discomfort while pursuing his long-term goals. However, it prevents him from creating unhealthy emotions such as depression and self-pity in his mind as such emotions weaken his capacity to deal with adverse conditions and events in his life. Even healthy negative emotions help him accept obnoxious facets of the world and life, try to change them if possible and lump with them without whining when they cannot be changed.

Ellis might have derived his philosophy of ULA partly from the writings of ancient and modern philosophers. He had partly started inventing and practising the rudiments of that philosophy since the age of 16. He claims that when he was just four years old, he had laid down some rules for himself. Following are those rules:

1. Life is full of hassles you can't control or eliminate.
2. Hassles are never terrible unless you make them so.
3. What does happen could always be worse.
4. Making a fuss about problems make them worse.

Dr Daniel N. Wiener (1988), the first biographer of Ellis, remarks that it is not easy to disapprove what Ellis claimed about his ability to think rationally even when he was a four-year-old boy. Moreover, Dr Wiener affirms that Ellis' brother Paul and his best friend Manny confirmed that he did think and behave as claimed by him even from his very young age. In this context, it is worth recalling that Ellis' mother called him 'a little human scientist' and 'quite a thinker' when he was a very young boy.

Unconditional Acceptance and Other Philosophies

Christian philosophy: Ellis was an atheist and secular humanist. Yet, he did not hesitate to admit that his philosophy of UOA comes quite closer to the Christian philosophy's cardinal principle, 'accept the sinner but not the sin'. Therefore, he did not find it difficult to agree with anyone who suggests that it would be useful to show to the Christian clients that the philosophy and actions of Jesus were similar to some basic tenets of REBT.

In his book, *Reason in Pastoral Counseling*, Dr Paul Hauck (1972) remarks that it is ironic that an atheist like Ellis offers a system of psychotherapy which, in some ways, is quite similar to Christian doctrine. Ellis agreed with Paul Hauck, but did not fail to point out that it is also ironic that the Christian doctrine, as well as the philosophy of many other religions, is so contradictory that it easily embraces unconditional forgiveness or grace and unconditional damnation and hell too!

Buddhism: In order to broaden the scope of REBT, Ellis started studying Buddhism in his later life. There were striking similarities in

REBT philosophy and Buddhist philosophy. The REBT concepts of others (UOA) and life (ULA) were very close to the concepts described by His Holiness Dalai Lama in his book, *The Art of Happiness: The Handbook for Living* (His Holiness the Dalai Lama, & Cutler, 1998). He illustrated variety of concepts in the book for how to ride through life's obstacles on a deep and abiding source of inner peace. The concept of unconditional acceptance is prominent among them. These concepts also show close proximity with the characteristics of a self-actualized person described in REBT, which we will see later in this chapter. In 2013, Susan Holt and Carol Austad (2013) published an article that explores conceptual and methodological similarities between REBT and Tibetan Buddhism and examines some of the values and concepts they share.

Unconditional Acceptance in Ellis' Personal Life

Earlier, we have seen how Ellis became a pacifist at the age of 15. One day after seeing a movie, he returned home and patched things up with his sister Janet by forgiving her for her nasty behaviour and accepting her unconditionally. Thus, the concept of UOA was incipient in his mind long before it took a concrete shape in his system of psychotherapy.

How is Ellis' own record in this respect, namely, accepting oneself unconditionally? Quite good, as can be gathered from the chapter, 'Nobody Need Feel Ashamed or Guilty About Anything', which he contributed to the book, *The Naked Therapist*, edited by Sheldon Kopp (1976).

In this chapter, Ellis described a serious mistake he made when he was a young therapist. Since he began to practise psychotherapy, he had decided not to socialize with his clients or their friends. Yet on one occasion, he committed the blunder of developing social and sexual relations with one Sarah who was a friend of his client, Josephine. Afterwards, Josephine herself overtly showed sexual interest in Ellis, but he sternly refused to have any relation with her. Unfortunately, she later found out about Ellis' relations with Sarah. As one can easily imagine, this created many complicated problems.

Ellis felt ashamed and guilty for what he had done, but managed to get rid of his emotional disturbance with the help of REBT. He also described how he could have thoroughly gotten rid of his emotional disturbance by learning to accept himself unconditionally although disapproving of his immoral behaviour.

In this connection, one may say that the fact Ellis had written about his moral lapse so candidly tends to show that he practised what he preached, namely, USA.

In this context, it may be interesting to note what Fredric B. Kleiner (1979) says in one of his articles. He endorses Ellis' suggestion that more researches may be conducted to test the hypothesis that a man can achieve USA by giving up rating his self or essence. However, he doubts the feasibility of doing such studies because he has never come across anyone who refrains from rating one's self. Even Ellis himself does not seem to have achieved this goal. Although, some Zen masters, yoga experts and Tibetan Lamas who also extol the advantages of not judging one's self or essence may be tested on this self-rating continuum.

Nevertheless, Ellis claimed that he began to teach his clients to forcefully dispute their musturbatory ideologies and dissociate themselves from their performances. He also claimed that he succeeded with 30 per cent of his clients at least to some extent.

Self-actualization

Imagine that Aditi, Vikram and Saniya chose to undergo psychotherapy by approaching Ellis. What line of treatment will Ellis adopt? Obviously, the final goal of Ellis would be to help them achieve their respective practical goal by overcoming their emotional disturbance which is compounding their practical problem. For instance, Ellis will help Aditi face the job interview by getting rid of her anxiety and also acquiring USA. He will help Vikram get along with his boss by overcoming his anger and also acquiring UOA. Finally, he will teach Saniya to follow the diet prescribed by her doctor by releasing herself from the clutches of handicapping depression and developing HFT.

Ellis has a second and a more comprehensive goal in his mind while treating his clients. He is not content with just helping his clients achieve better emotional health and live with less unhappiness. He aspires to encourage and teach his clients, and people who listen to his talks and read his books, to live more happy and productive life. Let us recall that Ellis was interested in philosophy, particularly philosophy of happiness, from the age of 16. He believed that when people relieve themselves of their burden of emotional disturbance, they can zestfully find and pursue their long-term goals, plans and values and thereby actualize their partly inborn and partly socially acquired potentialities. If they get absorbed in some self-chosen goals and values, they will feel happier and fulfilled.

Helping people achieve their potentialities and to self-actualization is not an easy task. It is beset with complicated problems. Many eminent psychologists such as Abraham Maslow and Carl Rogers as well as other social thinkers such as S.I. Hayakawa and Rollo May have expanded their views about tackling this complex issue. Few objections were raised on the self-actualization theories formulated by these above thinkers. Ellis took into consideration these objections and came up with his own views on these theories. Ellis believed that the goals of mental health and self-actualization are not completely identical. There is a large area of overlap between them. Therefore, the characteristics of self-actualizing persons described by Ellis include the characteristics of mentally healthy persons too.

He worked with Ted Crawford (Ellis, 1994; Ellis & Crawford, 2000; Ellis & Blau, 1998) for a number of years on his theory of self-actualization and its linkage with REBT. Both of them agreed on the following few important guidelines of self-actualization (Holt & Austad, 2013):

1. Actively choosing self-actualization
2. Disputing absolutistic *shoulds* and *musts* that blocks its achievement
3. Preferring, but not requiring, the solving of self-actualizing problems
4. Tolerance of oneself and others
5. Overcoming procrastination and LFT
6. Framing the problem as a systemic problem to be redesigned
7. Moving from either/ors towards and/alsos, including ambiguity, paradox, inconsistency and confusion and then working toward an integrated wholeness

The characteristics based on these guidelines are not completely different from those mentioned by Carl Rogers and Abraham Maslow. These characteristics also mirror the ideas of Alfred Korzybski, the founder, and S.I. Hayakawa, the promulgator of general semantics, a school of thought which significantly influenced REBT (Holt & Austad, 2013). The key characteristics of self-actualized people that are endorsed by Rogers, Maslow and general semantics and with which REBT agreed are summarized here.

1. **Self-awareness:** Self-actualizing people (SAPs) know and face their own feelings, whether they are positive or negative. When

they feel angry, hostile, anxious, panicky or depressed, they acknowledge these feelings, although they don't express these emotions in their day-to-day lives. Yet, they accept the fact that they are disturbed by those and similar other handicapping emotions. At the same time, they try to overcome those handicapping emotions as much as possible. Thus, they know themselves in the sense that they have a good insight into their emotional states. They also know how limited is their knowledge of themselves.

2. **Nonconformity and individualism:** SAPs strive to cultivate and preserve their individuality. They don't meekly conform to all the social and other norms of the group and culture in which they live. At the same time, they do not senselessly rebel against the social cultural norms just to prove their rebelliousness. They largely follow their own paths in love, sex, marital, vocational, recreational and other spheres of life.

3. **Acceptance of human animality:** SAPs accept the fact that they, like all human beings, have several obnoxious physical aspects and functions. They don't feel terribly disgusted with some unpleasant bodily products, functions, and odours of themselves and others. They accept such aspects of human beings as part of their biological and animal inheritance.

4. **Tolerance:** SAPs are flexible enough to recognize that there are similarities and differences in the world around them. Especially, they are not blind to the differences among things and people. They do not see all roses as red, all school hostels as temples peacefully and exclusively dedicated to learning or all experiments in art and literature as rubbish. As they are mentally flexible, they are willing to learn and grow in the multifaceted world in which they live. Similarly, being flexible in their thinking, they find it easy to follow Alfred Korzybski, the founder of general semantics, who is against labelling things as either/or and black or white. Rather, they are willing to view them in terms of both/and. For instance, people have good traits, bad traits and some of their traits are just neutral—neither good nor bad.

5. **Social interest and ethical trust:** Although SAPs believe in individualism and non-conformity, they are neither selfish nor antisocial. They are definitely ethical, trustworthy, constructive and socialized. They fully acknowledge being members of some society. Just as they work for self-interest, they also endeavour to further the interests of other people.

6. **Enlightened self-interest:** SAPs know that when they are good to others, they are best to themselves. Therefore, although they give the top priority to their self-interest, they do not deny the right of other people to work for their own interest. As a result, SAPs help other people achieve their goals. They know that in order to achieve their goals, they require the cooperation of other people. Moreover, the goal of their self-interest is enjoying themselves. Their focus is not on proving anything about themselves.

7. **Self-direction:** Although SAPs concentrate on pursuing their self-interest, as described previously, they follow the policy of enlightened self-interest. Therefore, they help others to fulfil their interests. To achieve their own goals, they mainly depend on their own resources and abilities. They do seek assistance of others and provide assistance to them. They largely depend on themselves for their effectiveness and well-being.

8. **Commitment and intrinsic enjoyment:** SAPs engage in different pursuits such as interesting work and sports because they find such activities enjoyable. Of course, they are not against achievement and success. Indeed, they do want to achieve and become successful in their lives. However, they involve themselves with some people, things and ideas because such involvements give them immense pleasure. When they are committed to some long-term and vitally absorbing interests, they feel fulfilled and happy.

9. **Creativity and originality:** As SAPs are not meek conformists, they are likely to find and follow a somewhat innovative approach to their goals and purposes. This increases the probability that their work and recreational pursuits are characterized by creativity and originality.

10. **Risk-taking and experimenting:** Practically, no one can be a self-actualizing person without taking risks and experimenting in various aspects of life. SAPs do not hesitate to experiment with many individuals and social activities. Naturally, they are not afraid of failing in certain tasks and even experiencing and suffering defeats. They survive such unpleasant adventures (or misadventures) and eventually discover better ways of enjoying life.

11. **Acceptance of ambiguity and uncertainty:** SAPs acknowledge that the world is full of ambiguity, uncertainty, the unknown, approximation and to some extent even disorder. Certainly, this is not the best of all possible worlds! The world in which we live

is characterized by probability and chance. Yet, SAPs believe that even such an imperfect world gives them the opportunity to learn, strive for something meaningful and thereby enjoy the process of living.

12. **Flexibility and scientific thinking:** One of the main principles of REBT is that human beings disturb themselves because they interpret and evaluate the happenings in their lives in the light of their rigid, inflexible and empirically untenable beliefs. They can reduce their emotional disturbance if they give up their dogmatic *musts* and *shoulds* and learn to live with more flexible and empirically verifiable beliefs. That is exactly what science advocates, namely, empirical verification or falsification of a hypothesis. Naturally, science disapproves rigidity and favours flexibility in thinking. The scientific approach teaches SAPs the philosophy of wanting various things in life, but not desperately insisting that their wants be fulfilled. Therefore, as followers of the scientific method, SAPs think and behave in a more reasonable manner in regards to their desires and goals.

13. **Long-range hedonism:** SAPs are not averse to seeking pleasures and enjoying life. Not only do they learn from Epictetus, but from Epicurus as well, who preached that seeking pleasures was natural and advisable. They do not succumb to the temptations of the moment which tend to destroy their pleasures, health and happiness in the long run. Rather, they focus on sanely enjoying themselves today and tomorrow as well. Thus, they intelligently enjoy their life for a long time rather than foolishly enjoying today and dying tomorrow.

14. **Unconditional acceptance of oneself and others:** SAPs unconditionally accept themselves and others. They evaluate their own performance without evaluating their totality. Similarly, they evaluate the performance of others without evaluating their totality. As a result, they are able to live and enjoy life without feeling too much anxiety, guilt, depression, anger, hostility, etc. Besides, this approach helps them look forward to zestfully involving themselves in creative pursuits.

15. **Work and practice:** As SAPs unconditionally accept themselves, they do not hesitate to accept the responsibility for their emotional disturbance. Therefore, when they are upset, they don't disown their responsibility by blaming others. They also admit that no

matter the cause of their childhood disturbance, they don't have to continue to remain victims of their childhood disturbance. They can learn to overcome their disturbance by work and practice. Even for behaving more effectively and living a happier life, they have to exert themselves. Nobody owes them happiness!

The description shows that REBT not only endorses self-actualizing philosophy, but describes a path of its attainment too.

References

Bertocci, P. (1963). *Personality and the Good: Psychological and Ethical Perspectives.* New York, NY: David Mckay.

Branden, N. (1970). *The Psychology of Self-Esteem.* New York, NY: Bantam.

Burns, D. (1985). *Intimate Connections: The Clinically Proven Programme for Making Close Friends and Finding a Loving Partner.* Signet, NY: New American Library.

Davis, J.W. (1972). *Value and Valuation: Axiological Studies in Honor of Robert Hartman.* Knoxville, Tennessee: University of Tennessee Press.

Ellis, A. (1968). *Is Objectivism a Religion?* New York, NY: Lyle Stuart. [Rev. ed. *Ayn Rand: Her Fascistic and Fanatically Religious Philosophy.*]

―――. (1971). *The Case Against Religion: A Psychotherapist's View.* New York: Institute for Rational Living.

―――. (1972). *Psychotherapy and the Value of a Human Being.* New York: Institute for Rational-Emotive Therapy. [Reprinted in Ellis. A., & Dryden, W. (1990). *The Essential Albert Ellis.* New York, NY: Springer.]

―――. (1973). Unhealthy love: Its causes and treatment. In M.E. Curtin (Ed.), *Symposium on Love* (pp. 175–97). New York, NY: Behavioural Publications. [Reprinted New York, NY: Institute for Rational-Emotive Therapy.]

―――. (1978). Atheism: A cure for neurosis. *American Atheist, 20*(3), 10–13.

―――. (1983). *The Case Against Religiosity.* New York, NY: Institute for Rational-Emotive Therapy.

―――. (1984). Rational-emotive therapy (RET) and pastoral counseling: A reply to Richard Wessler. *The Personnel and Guidance Journal, 62*(5): 266–67.

―――. (1993). The advantages and disadvantages of self-help therapy materials. *Professional Psychology: Research and Practice, 24*(3): 335–39.

―――. (1994). *Reason and Emotion in Psychotherapy. A Comprehensive Method of Treating Human Disturbances* (revised and updated, p. 393). New York, NY: Carol Publishing.

―――. (1997). Can counseling be Christian? *Christian Counselling Today, 5*(1), 48–49.

―――. (1999). *Make Yourself Happy and Remarkable Less Disturbable.* Mumbai: Jaico Publishing House.

Ellis, A. (2010). *All Out! Albert Ellis with Debbie Joffe Ellis: An Autobiography.* New York, NY: Prometheus Books.

Ellis, A., & Blau, S. (1998). *The Albert Ellis Reader: A Guide to Well-being Using Rational-Emotive Behaviour Therapy* (pp. 190–93) [A Citadel Press Book]. New York, NY: Carol Publishing.

Ellis, A., & Crawford, T. (2000). *Making Intimate Connections: 7 Guidelines for Great Relationships and Better Communication.* Atascadero, CA: Impact Publication.

Ellis, A., & Harper, R. (1975). *A New Guide to Rational Living* (p. 95). Modesto, CA: Melvin Powers.

Frankl, V. (1959). *Man's Search for Meaning.* New York, NY: Pocket Books.

Gandhi. M.K. (1984). *Anasaktiyoga: Translation in Gujarati of the Bhagavad Gita.* Ahmedabad: Navajivan Prakashan Mandir.

Grayling, A.C. (2004). *What Is Good?* (pp. 92–93). London: Phoenix.

Hartman, R.S. (1959). *The Measurement of Value.* Crotonville, NY: General Electric.

Hauck, P. (1972). *Reason in Pastoral Counseling.* Philadelphia, PA: Westminster Press.

His Holiness the Dalai Lama, & Cutler, H. (1998). *The Art of Happiness: The Handbook for Living.* New York, NY: Putnam Publishing Group.

Holt, S.A., & Austad, C.S. (2013). A comparison of rational emotive therapy and Tibetan Buddhism: Albert Ellis and the Dalai Lama. *International Journal of Behavioural Consultation and Therapy, 7*(4), 8–11.

Kleiner, Fredric B. (1979). Commentary on Albert Ellis' article. In A. Ellis & J. Whiteley (Eds.), *Theoretical and Empirical Foundations of Rational-Emotive Therapy.* California, CA: Brooks/Cole.

Kopp, S. (1976). *The Naked Therapist: A Collection of Embarrassments.* New York, NY: Cornell University.

Kwee, M., & Ellis, A. (1998). The interface between rational emotive behavior therapy (REBT) and Zen. *Journal of Rational-Emotive & Cognitive-Behaviour Therapy, 16*(1), 5–43.

May, R. (1967). *Psychology and the Human Dilemma.* Van Nostrand. [Rev. ed. (1996) New York: Norton.]

Newman, M., & Berkowitz, B. (1971). *How to be Your Own Best Friend?* New York, NY: Random House Publishing Group.

Nieslen, S.L., Johnson, W.B., & Ellis, A. (2001). *Counseling and Psychotherapy with Religious Persons: A Rational Emotive Behavior Therapy Approach.* Mahwah, NJ: Laurence Erlbaum Associates.

Phadke, K.M. (1968–2003). *Albert Ellis Papers* [Series I: Correspondence, 1947–2006], Correspondence of K.M. Phadke & Dr Albert Ellis, Columbia University Libraries Archival Collection. Retrieved from http://findingaids.cul.columbia.edu/ead/nnc-rb/ldpd_8683406/dsc/1

Pies, R. (2000). Symptoms, suffering, and psychodynamics: A personal journey from RET to the Talmud. *Voices, 36*(4), 61–72.

Rand, A., & Branden, N. (1964). *The Virtue of Selfishness: A New Concept of Egoism.* New York, NY: Penguin Books.

Rogers, C. (1961). *On Becoming A Person: A Therapist's View of Psychotherapy.* New York, NY: Houghton Mifflin Company. [Rev. ed. (1995). New York: Houghton Mifflin Company.]

Russell, B. (1930). *The Conquest of Happiness.* London: George Allen & Unwin.

Russell, B. (1946). *History of Western Philosophy*. London: George Allen & Unwin.

Wessler, R.L. (1984). A bridge too far: Incompatibilities of rational-emotive therapy and pastoral counseling. *The Personnel and Guidance Journal, 62*(7): 264–66.

Wiener, D.N. (1988). *Albert Ellis: Passionate Skeptic*. New York, NY: Praeger.

Further Readings

Ellis, A. (1978). Atheism: A cure for neurosis. *American Atheist, 20*(3), 10–13.

———. (1988). Comments on Sandra Warnock's 'rational-emotive therapy and the Christian client'. *Journal of Rational-Emotive & Cognitive-Behavior Therapy, 7*(4), 275–77.

———. (1992a). Do I really hold that religiousness is irrational and equivalent to emotional disturbance? *American Psychologist, 47*(3), 428–29.

———. (1992b). My current views on rational-emotive therapy (RET) and religiousness. *Journal of Rational-Emotive & Cognitive-Behavior Therapy, 10*(1), 37–40.

Phadke, K.M. (1999). *Adhunik Sanjivani*. Mumbai: Tridal Prakashan.

8

Therapeutic Process of REBT

When Ellis hoisted the flag of rebellion by presenting the paper 'Rational Psychotherapy' at the Annual Convention of APA in Chicago on 31 August 1956, he mainly focused on describing how the system of psychotherapy invented by him was different from the highly respected therapies prevailing at that time. Similarly, in the subsequent introductory presentations of his psychotherapeutic system, he continued to highlight how it was to be distinguished from other popular therapies.

Although, many aspects of his newly invented therapy were also similar to those of other therapies, he did not bother delineating them. Later, he and some of his followers showed dissimilarities as well as similarities between their therapy and other therapies. Keeping this in mind, in this chapter, we shall outline the therapeutic process of REBT, which we bifurcate into its characteristics, goals and insights.

First, we consider different characteristics of therapeutic process such as its active-directive approach, therapeutic relationship, the attributes of effective therapist and the phases and steps of therapeutic interventions. Second, we review its goals and insights.

Characteristics of Therapeutic Process

Active-Directive Therapeutic Approach

REBT is one of the pioneering psychotherapies of advocating active-directive therapeutic approach. To be precise, an REBT therapist actively directs the client to detect the irrational philosophic basis of his psychological disturbance and teaches him how he can examine, challenge and replace it with an alternative rational philosophy. This is avowedly an educational process which continues until the client learns to be his own therapist in the future.

REBT is distinctively different in this feature from other schools of psychotherapy as they advocate non-directive therapeutic approach. In this approach, the therapist's role is relatively passive and he is expected not to intertwine the client's process of exploration. Therefore, more time and space is given to the client to work out his own solutions.

While commenting on this approach, Ellis mentioned that during a therapeutic session, the client is emotionally disturbed whereas the therapist is not. Hence, the therapist is in a better state of mind to direct the client actively in the course of the therapy. Ellis assumed that clients would be helped more effectively if the therapist is active and directive. Especially, at the beginning of a therapeutic session, the REBT therapist quickly and directly helps the client identify the philosophic causes of his disturbance and his dysfunctional behaviour. Similarly, he does not spend any time on reviewing the childhood experiences of the client.

This style of working with the client is a logical corollary of the $A \times B = C$ theory of emotional disturbance. If the client is emotionally disturbed at a given time, it is because he is doggedly clinging to some irrational beliefs at that very time. Therefore, the therapist aims at detecting the current irrational beliefs of the client and then substituting those beliefs by alternative rational beliefs. Since the client has been attached to his irrational beliefs strongly and for a longer duration, the therapist goes about achieving his aim energetically and forcefully. The therapist launches a concerted, forceful and energetic attack on the irrational beliefs of the client. However, he takes care to see that he only attacks the client's irrational beliefs and not the client himself.

There is another reason why Ellis used force and energy while helping the client get rid of his irrational beliefs. The therapist, who uses a very mild and gentle style of changing the client's irrational beliefs, may help the client acquire an intellectual insight into his problems. For example, the client may superficially or lightly understand that his current beliefs are irrational and it would be better to abandon them and imbibe alternative rational beliefs, instead. This sort of a mild and superficial understanding is not enough to rigorously motivate him to actively work at bringing about a desired change in his irrational beliefs because his conviction about his deeply held beliefs is still too strong.

On the contrary, a therapist who adopts a forceful and energetic style not only helps the client to acquire intellectual insight but also emotional insight into his problems. In other words, his conviction about the utility of rational beliefs and the futility of his irrational beliefs becomes too strong. As a result, he becomes emotionally charged to work at changing his irrational beliefs and dysfunctional behaviour.

In *Reasons and Emotions in Psychotherapy*, Ellis (1994, pp. 221–23) had mentioned 18 reasons of adopting active-directive approach. Some of the reasons are as follows:

1. People cling to irrational beliefs very strongly and rigidly. Therefore, vigorous persuasion of the therapist is needed so that they can give up those beliefs.
2. As an REBT therapist doesn't need the clients' approval for effective therapy, he can directly go after client's nonsense and try to help them change it.
3. Resistance to change is very strong in disturbed clients. Hence, REBT therapists work quite hard to help clients overcome this resistance.
4. People's triple-headed indoctrination with irrational beliefs—from their parents, society and their own creation—makes their *musts* very strong. They not only creatively construct their absolutistic *musts* but they constructively continue to upset themselves with the same basic *musts*. Hence, active-directive and sometimes forceful therapy is required to work on them.
5. REBT therapists work with ABC structure which consists of identifying and challenging irrational beliefs and hence, they have to be alert and watchful for specific cues to these beliefs. For example, key words, phrases, intonations, non-verbal behaviour, etc. The therapists try not to let these slip by unattended, by becoming directive (Walen, DiGiuseppe, & Wessler, 1980).

REBT therapist using active directive therapeutic approach shows the two characteristics mentioned here.

1. **Directiveness:** An REBT therapist is directive in his style in the sense that he knows where the process will lead towards and gives the directions accordingly. An REBT therapist does not wait for the client's realization on his own problem solving but he directs him to the path and helps him as concretely as possible. REBT provides flexibility concerning how much direction *should* be provided at any point in the therapeutic process (Dryden, 1994).

   An REBT therapist is directive in assessment and interventions by providing the structure to the therapy. In the non-directive approach, the therapy is usually unstructured as clients explore the process gradually, something which cannot be predetermined. In REBT sessions, the process can be outlined beforehand. The client is given a choice to choose his own problem to work on and the ABC structure is used for the assessment and intervention. The REBT therapist is highly directive in using the ABC structure in the following three steps.

(i) *Focusing on 'C'*—Therapist provides help to the client in identifying self-defeating emotions.

(ii) *Identifying correct 'A'*—Therapist actively guides the client to search which aspect of 'A' has triggered 'C'.

(iii) Working on 'B'—Therapist assists the client to make him aware about B–C connection. During the intervention, the therapist actively teaches the client the disputation of irrational beliefs. Gaining insights on rational beliefs and replacing them in the place of irrational beliefs is the last part of this structure.

However, these steps are not rigid. Each therapist can vary the amount of structure or can adopt it to his own style and can modify it if required.

2. **Activeness:** An REBT therapist actively teaches the clients various methods of problem solving in the following mentioned ways.

(i) *Hypothetical-educative approach*—As DiGiuseppe (1991) suggested REBT therapists follow hypothetical-deductive approach. It includes building the hypotheses about the client's irrational beliefs and verifying them by asking his own feedback. By using this approach, not only the therapist but also the client becomes active and participative. A number of questions are asked to the clients such as

- Socratic questions. To encourage the client to think for himself and guide him for problem solving.
- Disputation questions. To challenge the irrational beliefs by using three criteria—factual, functional and logical.

(ii) *Educational approach*—As REBT uses an educational approach to the therapy, it provides teaching opportunities at various stages of assessment and interventions. REBT uses didactic explanations. These explanations are provided to the client by using didactic methods such as ABC framework or client's role in the therapeutic process.

At this juncture, it is interesting to know the comments of Ellis' co-therapists on his active-directive style. They (Walen, DiGiuseppe & Wessler, 1980) described that because of Ellis' directive style, the group members frequently reported feelings of warmth and respect towards Ellis. They also reported that he demonstrated his caring by asking many questions, his complete attention to their problems, his advocating of an accepting and tolerant philosophy and teaching them something immediate that they could do to reduce their pain. This description reveals how active directive style helps to develop rapport-building quickly and effectively.

However, it is not necessary that all REBT practitioners have to follow the active-directive, energetic and forceful style of Ellis. Some therapists prefer to be more passive and gentle with their clients. With some clients, Ellis' forceful style even proved to be counterproductive. It is then obvious that the therapist has to use his judgment and adopt a suitable style while working with different clients.

Therapeutic Relationship

Teaching skills: The therapist works with the client just as a teacher works with a student. Hence, the therapist is required to possess, besides a sound knowledge of REBT, good teaching skills. He behaves authoritatively with the client, but ensures that his style of teaching is not authoritarian. He is not supposed to establish any specific relationship with the client. Of course, he is considerate and humane with the clients. Yet, he is flexible enough to vary his method of relating to his clients when he considers it necessary.

A distinguishing feature of the relationship between the therapist and the client in REBT is that the therapist is a concerned professional but does not offer excessive warmth to the client because of two reasons. First, if the therapist expresses too much warmth and support, the client's need for love and approval may be reinforced. Perhaps, the client who receives excessive warmth and support from the therapist may show improvement in his emotional disturbance and dysfunctional behaviour for a wrong reason. This kind of improvement could be a result of getting what he believes he *must* have—approval and support. If so, his improvement is deceptive as it is a spin-off of getting his irrational philosophy of life reinforced.

Second, if the therapist shows too much of warmth and support, the client's faulty philosophy of LFT may get reinforced. Usually clients already have LFT; therefore, they always ask for other people's assistance for managing their day-to-day problems. Hence, if the therapist is too kind and supportive, clients' irrational belief that they need the help of others gets strengthened.

Unconditional acceptance: One of the major objectives of a therapist is to teach the client to accept himself unconditionally, irrespective of bad or self-defeating behaviour. In other words, the client is taught what is called USA in REBT. When the client learns this lesson, he would be able to rate his thoughts, feelings and acts, good or bad without considering himself a good or bad person. He accepts himself as a unique but fallible human being who behaves in many useful ways.

In order to facilitate this process of teaching unconditional acceptance, the therapist himself accepts the client unconditionally without labelling him as good or bad. Although, he does not fail to notice that, at certain times, his clients behave in a self-defeating manner both in the therapy sessions and outside. He may even draw his client's attention to his self-defeating behaviour which may retard the progress and purpose of therapeutic sessions.

Before Ellis invented this therapy, the field of psychotherapy had been largely influenced by Carl Rogers' theory and practice of counselling. According to Carl Rogers (1942), three conditions are necessary for bringing about the desired therapeutic changes in the client. These three conditions are fulfilled by the therapist when he shows empathy, genuineness and unconditional positive regard to his client. Whereas, Ellis believes that there are no such conditions for doing effective therapy. All that is required is that somehow the client reviews and changes his faulty attitudes or philosophy of life and then learns to adopt rational attitudes or philosophy of life. He can do so with or without the help of a therapist or for that matter, any outside source.

However, Ellis agrees that the three conditions laid down by Carl Rogers facilitate the therapeutic process, providing they are adopted with some modifications. As regards to the condition of genuineness, even any modification is not required because the genuineness of the therapist facilitates the therapeutic process. When the therapist conducts sessions with the client, he feels free to talk about how he solves certain problems in his life. If the client asks him questions about his personal life, he frankly answers those questions. Of course, on such occasions, he does not fail to use his discretion. In this way, he is therapeutically genuine in dealing with the client.

In the previous chapter, we have seen that Ellis is somewhat sceptical about showing unconditional positive regard to the client. In his view, it creates a belief in the client's mind that he is good or respectable as his therapist shows unconditional regard to him. Thus, he may unwittingly learn CSA. In this way, the client becomes dependent on the therapist in order to consider himself worthwhile. Whereas, the aim of therapy is to help him accept himself just because he is a unique human being; however, being fallible, some of his acts are good and noble, but some are bad and ignoble.

In view of this disadvantage of showing unconditional positive regard to the client, Ellis recommends that the therapist had better accept his client unconditionally. This is what is called UOA in REBT. This kind of the therapist's behaviour facilitates the process of helping the client become self-dependent and unconditionally accept himself whether or not he achieves success and other people's appreciation.

Philosophic empathy: As regard to the third condition laid down by Carl Rogers, namely, empathy, Ellis has no quarrel. Usually, when the therapist shows empathy to the client, he communicates his understanding of how the client feels. This is called affective empathy. In REBT, the therapist offers this kind of empathy to the client. However, he goes a step further and offers philosophic empathy.

The concept of philosophic empathy has its origin in one of the main principles of REBT which states that the client's disturbing feelings are largely caused by his irrational philosophy of life. When the therapist understands the client's disturbing feelings, he quickly infers the irrational philosophic basis of those feelings. He then tells the client that he has identified the faulty philosophy underlying his emotional disturbance.

Humour in therapy: According to Ellis, one reason why clients become emotionally disturbed is that they take themselves, their problems, the people around them and the world in which they live too seriously. This is largely a result of their musturbatory and grandiose beliefs. Therefore, the therapist shows the client that it is advantageous to be serious but not too serious about life. To bring home to the client this idea, the therapist injects generous doses of humour into his therapeutic sessions. However, he ensures that the target of his humour is foolish thoughts, feelings and actions of the client and never the client himself.

The purpose of humorous interventions is to puncture the client's musturbatory and grandiose outlook on life. In order to achieve this objective more dramatically, Ellis even sings rational humorous songs composed by him, which were published in the book *A Garland of Rational Songs* (Ellis, 1977). These songs humorously express the message that 'if you don't develop a good sense of humour, you will develop an emotional tumour'. This slogan is created by Ellis himself! Box 8.1 presents an example of rational humorous song composed by Ellis.

Box 8.1

Example of a Rational Humorous Song

WHINE, WHINE, WHINE!

(Tune: Yale Whiffenpool Song. By Guy Scull–A Harvard Man!)
I cannot have all of my wishes filled...
Whine, Whine, Whine!
I cannot have every frustration stilled...
Whine, Whine, Whine!
Life really owes me the things I miss,
Fate has to grant me eternal bliss!
And since I *must* settle for less than this...
Whine, Whine, Whine!

— Dr Albert Ellis

Source: Ellis (1999, p. 141).

Focus on emotional problems: Normally, people choose to undergo psychotherapy because they are confronted with two types of problems. First, they want to tackle some practical problems in their lives. For example, Aditi may want to learn some techniques of giving a good job interview. Vikram may want to learn good interpersonal skills so that he can deal with his boss effectively and Saniya may be eager to learn a method of implementing the diet prescribed by her doctor. People who choose to undergo psychotherapy are also confronted with the second type of problems, namely, the emotional disturbances which they themselves create about their practical problems. Their self-created emotional problems compound and complicate their first type of problems, namely, their practical problems.

The therapist, who follows REBT, will begin by focusing on the second type of problems (emotional problems) of clients. For instance, he will help Aditi, Vikram and Saniya to first get rid of their unhealthy emotions of anxiety, anger and depression respectively. His assumption is that when human beings learn to reduce the disturbance created by their unhealthy emotions, they can harness their inborn intelligence and acquired knowledge and skills to solve their practical problems more effectively.

On the contrary, if the therapist teaches some effective techniques of giving a good job interview to Aditi, interpersonal skills to Vikram and workable method of implementing the prescribed diet to Saniya, he will overlook his main task of detecting and changing the irrational beliefs underlying his client's faulty philosophies of life. As a result, his clients, though better equipped to tackle their problems, may continue to be susceptible to become emotionally upset when confronted with similar problems in the future.

That is the reason why the REBT practitioner makes it first to concentrate on helping the clients change their faulty philosophies of life which underlie their emotional disturbances. He then may teach them some techniques or skills to solve their practical problems. Thus, REBT is more depth-centred than therapies that focus on teaching some techniques and skills to the clients.

Effective REBT Therapist

What are the qualities required to become an effective REBT practitioner? A very general answer to this question is that a therapist who finds REBT's scientific and humanistic approach to life worthy of adopting and practising in his own life is more likely to become a competent REBT practitioner.

There exists hardly any empirical research on the characteristics of an effective REBT therapist. However, the REBT theory proposes a number of hypotheses (Ellis & Dryden, 1997) about some desirable attributes of the effective therapist. According to these hypotheses, the therapist will be called effective if he has following characteristics:

1. He is in tune with REBT philosophy.
2. He has practised REBT principles in his everyday life.
3. His worth is not involved in his client's improvement.
4. He doesn't need client's approval for therapeutic success.
5. He demonstrates and practices the philosophy of HFT.
6. He unconditionally accepts himself and clients as fallible human beings and does not put label as good or bad.

In addition, it is expected that the REBT practitioner does not hang on to any musturbatory ideology about himself, other people and the world in which he lives. To be more specific, he does not adhere to the following mentioned beliefs (Phadke & Khear, 1998), which adversely influence his effectiveness as a therapist:

1. I *must* be *always* successful with *every* client. (Musturbatory Ideology 1)

2. I *must* be a great therapist compared to other so-called well-known therapists. (Musturbatory Ideology 1)
3. My clients *must* appreciate all my efforts I put for their improvement. (Musturbatory Ideology 2)
4. Because I work so assiduously to help my clients, they also *must* work hard to improve themselves. (Musturbatory Ideology 2)
5. I am also a human being, and therefore, when I work as a therapist, I *must* enjoy my work and get *complete* satisfaction. (Musturbatory Ideology 3)
6. The therapy I use for my clients is not only beneficial to them but *must* benefit me too. (Musturbatory Ideology 3)

All these aspects of the therapist's personality present a model of a mentally healthy person before the client and thereby facilitate the therapeutic process.

The Phases of Therapeutic Interventions

When an REBT practitioner is all set to conduct the first therapeutic session, how does he begin to communicate with the client? Of course, first he greets the client and makes him feel comfortable and relaxed. Then he begins to explore how much the client knows about psychotherapy in general and REBT in particular. In the light of this kind of discussion, the therapist tries to understand what the client expects to happen in the process of therapy. If necessary, the therapist may even give a short lecture on the nature and goals of REBT.

In this way, the therapist helps the client decide the goal (G). In REBT, the goal (G) is usually two-fold. First, to reduce the client's emotional disturbance and make him feel better. Second, to help him get better by bringing about the desired change in his behaviour. These goals are achieved in three phases of therapeutic intervention. Each therapeutic session lasts for approximately 45 minutes. The numbers of sessions required for each phase is not fixed, but the outcome of each phase is more or less uniform in all therapeutic interventions.

1. **The initial phase:** When a client meets the therapist for individual therapy, the first step is a rapport building. By building good rapport with the client, the therapist encourages him to talk more about his concerns and helps him to feel at ease. The therapist explains to the

client the help he will get from the therapeutic sessions and asks him to communicate his expectations. He makes him aware if the expectations are unrealistic and helps him to set realistic goals of the session.

When the client narrates his current problem(s), the therapist does not bother to jot down the client's past. Nor does he use any diagnostic test to assess the client's problem(s). However, he may ask the client to fill in some kind of a biographical information form in order to collect the background information necessary to offer him therapy. Ellis believed that the best way to diagnose the client's problem(s) is to begin the therapy. The client's reactions in the first few therapeutic sessions reveal more about him than any psychological test.

When Ellis began practising REBT in this way, he initiated a rebellion against the established method of offering therapy to clients. Until then (and even now in some types of psychotherapies), the client's history was considered extremely important in therapy. In REBT, spending time for doing a historical analysis of the client's problem is considered unnecessary, distracting and sidestepping. Hence, the therapist directs the client to state the problem briefly.

The ABC framework is introduced to the client at this phase. The therapist breaks down the client's problem into three parts—activating event (A) beliefs (Bs) and emotional and behavioural consequences (Cs). The therapist's main focus is on the client's irrational beliefs (IBs) or his musturbatory ideologies. There are a number of ways of revealing this to the client. One of the ways is to demonstrate 10 different consequences (C) shown by 10 different people if they experience the same 'A' as client's. The therapist clarifies the doubts and queries of the client in an open and non-defensive manner. This phase generally ends when the client takes responsibility for self-change.

2. **The middle phase:** During this phase, the client is made aware of the existence of the irrational beliefs behind emotional disturbance. Since REBT's theory of emotional disturbance, namely, $A \times B = C$, states that human beings largely disturb themselves by their irrational or musturbatory ideologies, the therapy is mainly directed at substituting those irrational or musturbatory ideologies with alternative rational ideologies.

At this phase, the therapist has two tasks. First, identifying the client's irrational beliefs and second, disputing them vigorously (D).

Hence, the therapist tries to attack the client's core irrational belief and the alternative rational belief which could replace it. Both of these work together towards strengthening rational beliefs and weakening irrational beliefs. The therapist emphasizes on the current origin of the beliefs and does not invest therapeutic time in the search of the historical origin of these beliefs. Extensive work is done on the disputation of irrational beliefs. The therapist uses various therapeutic techniques at this phase to help the client. Some practitioners (Grieger & Boyd, 1980) stated that, in the middle phase of REBT intervention, the therapist helps the clients to work through his or her emotional and behavioural problems and to achieve the REBT re-education.

3. **The end phase:** This phase generally begins when the client shows considerable progress. The therapist makes it clear to the client that for bringing about the necessary changes in him, he will be required to participate actively in the process of change. His active participation will include, among other things, doing the assignments given to him.

   By this phase, the REBT philosophy is well internalized by the client. He not only becomes empowered to solve his own problems, but he is also ready to face future difficulties without the assistance of the therapist. At this stage, the client develops effective philosophy of life (E). The attainment of 'E' is followed by the termination and follow-up sessions.

Sometimes, in the very first session, the therapist offers the client some hypotheses which are likely to be at the root of his emotional and behavioural disturbance. The important point is that, in REBT, assessment of the client's problem is concurrent with the therapeutic process. There is no hard and fast rule that the therapist *must* first assess client's problem(s) and then begin the therapeutic process. On the contrary, the therapist is free to go ahead with therapy and change his assessment of the client if it is necessary to do so.

Feeling better and getting better: REBT makes a distinction between the two terms—'feeling better' and 'getting better'. Helping people get better rather than merely feel better is one of the key factors in REBT (Ellis, 1972). One of the Ellis' books (Ellis, 2001) is especially devoted to describe the difference between these two terms. Ellis said that it is a difference between what merely sounds good (feeling better) and what actually works (getting better). In short, the difference can be described as follows:

- *Feeling better*—It includes helping the client to reduce the disturbance and to make him feel better. It also involves a cessation of symptoms, and it works for a short period of time.
- *Getting better*—It is usually difficult to achieve. It involves not only a cessation of symptoms but also a philosophical insight into the human disturbance. It brings a long-term change in client's behaviour.

In the initial phases of therapeutic intervention, the therapist emphasizes on feeling better but as the intervention progresses, the client is expected to move towards getting better. Box 8.2 shows the summary (Dryden & Branch, 2008) of the therapeutic interventions in three phases.

Box 8.2

Summary of Therapeutic Interventions in Three Phases

The initial phase
To Establish a therapeutic alliance
To Socialize the client with REBT   } **Feeling Better**
Begin to assess and intervene target problem
Teach the ABCs of REBT
Deal with your client's doubts

The middle phase
Follow through on target problem
Encourage the client to engage in relevant tasks
Identify and challenge your client's core irrational beliefs
Deal with obstacles to change
Encourage the client to maintain and enhance gains
Undertake relapse prevention and deal with vulnerability factors
Encourage your client to become his own counsellor

The end phase
Decide on when and how to end
Encourage the client to summarize what has been learned   } **Getting Better**
Attribute improvement to client's efforts
Deal with obstacles to ending
Agree on criteria for follow-ups and for resuming therapy

The Steps in the Therapeutic Process

Ellis had mentioned (Ellis et al., 2003, p. 41) 13 sequential steps in the REBT therapeutic process. These steps help the client and the therapist to review the progress and provide the client the opportunity to revise his takeaway from the session. It also provides a checklist for the therapist to inspect the points he may have missed or overlooked. Box 8.3 presents the 13 steps of the REBT counselling process.

Box 8.3

Rational Emotive Behaviour Sequence

Step 1. Ask for a problem

Step 2. Define and agree upon the target problem

Step 3. Assess C

Step 4. Assess A

Step 5. Identify and assess any secondary emotional problems

Step 6. Teach the B–C connection

Step 7. Assess beliefs

Step 8. Connect irrational beliefs and C

Step 9. Dispute irrational beliefs (D)

Step 10. Prepare your client to deepen conviction in rational beliefs (E)

Step 11. Encourage your client to put new learning into practice

Step 12. Check homework assignments

Step 13. Facilitate the working through process

Case 8.1

Case of Suraj

Suraj is a 25-year-old man. When he met the therapist, he was disturbed due to a parking lot dispute he had with his neighbour a few days ago. Suraj does not have parking slots in his building premises. Those who own vehicles have to park their vehicles on the road. On road slots are not reserved for any specific vehicle and owners have to keep their eyes on the empty slots and have to step in quickly to capture it. In the last week, when Suraj was parking his vehicle in an empty slot, his neighbour arrived there in his vehicle. He started yelling at Suraj that the slot belonged to him as he parks his vehicle there every day and that Suraj needed to park at some other slot. This led to a heated argument between the two. At last, Suraj shifted his vehicle to another slot which was one kilometre away from his building.

Analysis of Case 8.1 in Reference to the Therapeutic Steps

Let us see how an REBT therapist deals with Suraj's disturbance and how he follows the steps of therapeutic process in the session. Here is the excerpt of the verbatim dialogue between Suraj and the therapist during the session. The relevant steps and important points of the therapeutic process are mentioned in the bracket in italics.

Therapist: What can I do for you?
(It is an opening statement of the session. Refers to Step 1, i.e., Ask for a problem.)

Suraj: I am disturbed.

Therapist: May I know what kind of disturbance you have?
(The therapist is moving the conversation towards Step 2, i.e., Define and agree upon the target problem.)

Suraj: I am experiencing anxiety, anger, resentment and rage.
(Refers to Step 3, i.e., Assess C)

Therapist: Good that you are aware of your disturbance. Which one is the most disturbing?
(The first statement shows that the therapist is acknowledging Suraj's emotions. Small compliments are needed to open up the discussion. The question indicates Step 3, i.e., Assess C. Here the therapist is using the active-directive approach. He is directing Suraj to move from a broad term of disturbance to a specific kind of emotional disturbance.)

Suraj: Rage.

Therapist: Rage is actually anger. It is intense anger. Never mind. I will go by your terminology. We will consider rage is your prominent emotion. Will you describe any recent incident when you experienced rage?
(The first statement shows that the therapist is probing further Step 3, i.e., Assess C. It shows that the therapist should have a good knowledge of emotions and their components. Next two statements are empathetic statements. The therapist is showing an agreement with Suraj's emotions. He is not putting his own words or terminology in Suraj's mouth. The role of empathy in therapeutic process is evident here. The last statement refers to Step 4, i.e., Assess A.)

Suraj: I had a fight with my neighbour over a parking slot. We do not have parking slots in our building premises. We have to park our vehicles on the road. Last week, when I was parking my vehicle in an empty slot, my neighbour arrived in his vehicle and started yelling at me that I *should* move to another slot as that slot belonged to him and he had to park his vehicle there. I was angry as on-road slots are not reserved for anybody. How can he demand the place just because he parks there every day? Finally, I parked my vehicle in another distant slot. I am disturbed because I feel that I *should* have done more.
(Description of A and C—Helping the therapist to reach Step 4, i.e., Assess A.)

Therapist: Let me summarize what you said. When you were parking your vehicle in an empty slot on the road, your neighbour arrived and demanded that it was his slot and you *should* shift your vehicle to another spot. You kept quiet and moved your vehicle to another distant slot. Now you feel that you *should* have done more. Have I understood correctly?
(Rephrasing and rechecking are important steps in the therapeutic process, which are evident in these sentences.)

Suraj: No, I didn't keep quiet. I argued with him. But now I feel that that was insufficient. I *should* have done more.

Therapist: Alright! You did take some measures, but you feel that they were insufficient. I *should* have done more. Will you tell me how you felt at that time?
(The therapist is rephrasing again. He is flexible in correcting the activating event [Step 4]. The question in the last statement shows that he is moving to Step 5, i.e., Identify and assess any secondary emotional problems.)

Suraj: I felt very small because I did something insufficient.

Therapist: Yes, which other ideas passed your mind? There *must* have been a flood of ideas. The event is still lingering in your mind. What have you imagined? What did you think?
(The therapist is leading the conversation towards Step 6, i.e., Teach the B–C connection. Identifying self-talk is an important step in B–C connection.)

Suraj: I felt worthless.

(Refers to Step 5 again, i.e., Identify and assess any secondary emotional problems. Suraj added one more emotion of worthlessness.)

Therapist: Alright! You felt worthless. Feel free to tell me about any other emotion that you felt.

(As Suraj added one more emotion, the therapist went back to Step 3, i.e., Assess C, and started collecting C again. The therapist is tolerant and he is giving flexibility to Suraj to add any emotion. The role of empathy in the therapeutic process is evident here once again.)

Suraj: ....

Therapist: Anything else that you felt?

(Therapist is collecting C to confirm Step 3, i.e., Assess C.)

Suraj: No.

(Step 3 completed. The therapist can move ahead.)

Therapist: Let me check what I can do for you. I can't go to your neighbour and tell him to stop abusing you over the parking slot, but I can help you manage your current emotion.

(The therapist is focusing on the current emotion and drawing Suraj's attention from A to B. He is precise in describing what he can do and what he cannot. This is an important step in goal setting.)

Suraj: Yes.

Therapist: You said that you *should* have done more. What prevented you from doing it?

(The therapist is taking the conversation towards Step 7, i.e., Assess belief. He has built up a hypothesis about Suraj's 'must', and he is verifying it by asking more questions. The use of the hypothetical educative approach is clearly seen here.)

Suraj: I thought that if I did something more, it would further provoke him and a new calamity would result.

Therapist: Ok. So you have not opted for that choice. Now, you are disturbed because you think that you *should* have done more. Can you tell me why you *should have done* something?

(Refers to Step 8, i.e., Connect irrational beliefs and C)

Suraj: ....

Therapist: Do you know the meaning of '*should*'? I will show you the meaning of '*should*'. (*The therapist holds pen in his hand.*) See this pen. What will happen if I remove my fingers?

Suraj: It will fall down due to a gravitational force.

Therapist: It '*should*' fall down. Here '*should*' is correct because the pen is non-living. It does not have any choice. Is this true with you too? Can you make this compulsion to human beings? Is there any force (like gravitational force) in your tongue that says that you '*should*' have talked?

(*This dialogue refers to Step 9, i.e., Dispute irrational beliefs (D). In the first part of the dialogue, the therapist is disputing 'must' emotively and vigorously with a live example. Because of the live example, Suraj gets reinforced to answer the question. In the last part of the dialogue, therapist is disputing logically.*)

Suraj: Yes, I understand. It would be better if I had talked.

Therapist: What is the difference between '*should* have' and 'could be better'?

(*Step 9, i.e., Dispute irrational beliefs, continues.*)

Suraj: In '*should*', there is compulsion and in better, it is not.

Therapist: You are saying that you '*should*' have done more. Actually, you have not done so. The event is over now. Is it realistic to say that I *should* have done more when actually you have not done so? Suppose I say that water *should* not be wet, when in reality it is wet. But I continue to say that it '*should*' not be wet, will it be realistic?

(*The therapist is disputing empirically and emotively with an example. He is moving towards Step 10, i.e., Prepare your client to deepen conviction in rational beliefs (E).*)

Suraj: No.

Therapist: You have no choice over whatever has happened. You have a choice for your future actions. If you continue to think that it would be better if I had talked, what will happen?

(*The first statement shows that the therapist is helping Suraj focus on the current state and is showing him that he still has a choice. In the next statement, the therapist is showing Suraj the benefits of giving up 'must'. Step 10, i.e., Prepare your client to deepen conviction in rational beliefs (E), completed.*)

Suraj: I will feel better.

Therapist: To strengthen this feeling, I will suggest you homework. Go home and write down three realistic steps which you will take up if the same incident happens in the future. It will prepare you in advance to face the situation. *(Refers to the Step 11, i.e., Encourage your client to put new learning into practice.)*

Suraj: I will certainly do it.

Therapist: Good! Tell me honestly, what are you feeling right now?

Suraj: More relaxed.

(In the next session, the therapist will deal with Suraj's other musturbatory ideologies such as 'my neighbour should not have done so'. He will follow Step 12 by checking the homework assignment given to Suraj and in further sessions, he will facilitate the working through process, i.e., Step 13.)

Elegant and Inelegant REBT

In many respects, REBT shows similarity to CBT or cognitive behaviour modification (Ellis, Young & Lockwood, 1987). But it also differs from these therapies in various aspects. The most important distinctive feature of REBT which clearly holds it apart from CBT is its elegant or preferential form. Ellis (1979) mentioned the two different forms of REBT intervention.

1. **Elegant or preferential REBT:** This is also called classical REBT. Bringing about a profound philosophical change in the client's assumptions is the distinguishing feature of elegant REBT. Here, the therapist not only works to improve the client's cognitive distortions but he also tries to change his fundamental dysfunctional philosophy. Elegant REBT teaches the client a more logico-empirical, problem-solving manner and uses disputation as one of its important therapeutic intervention. Elegant therapeutic intervention does not focus merely on symptom removal but provides coping strategies that clients can use to deal with a wide number of similar problems. It thus minimizes their chances of creating new emotional disturbances in the future. This intervention aims at the client's long-term improvement.

2. **General or inelegant REBT:** This form of REBT intervention is called inelegant as it does not bring a major philosophical change.

It may provide a coping strategy for existing emotional disturbance, but it cannot be applied to wide range of similar problems. It aims at a more symptomatic change. General REBT is more or less synonymous with CBT. It tries to improve dysfunctional thoughts or faulty cognitions by cognitive restructuring or reattribution or other similar techniques. It helps the client develop alternative ways of thinking and behaving which aims at reducing emotional disturbance.

Elegant REBT is invariably done as part of general or inelegant REBT. However, the reverse is not true.

Therapeutic Goals and Insights

Therapeutic Goals

We have studied what makes people disturbed and how their emotional disturbance leads them to behave in self-defeating ways. We also know the characteristics of emotionally healthy, happy people engaged in the pursuit of self-actualization.

The goals of REBT almost logically flow from its theoretical framework. Ellis (1967) further shows how REBT particularly stresses some goals.

1. **First goal:** The first goal of REBT is to help people reduce their unhealthy emotional upsets. This will certainly make people feel better. However, we have seen earlier that Ellis makes a distinction between feeling better and getting better. Making people just feel better is not the only goal of REBT. Usually, emotional disturbance of people makes them behave in dysfunctional, self-defeating ways. Therefore, REBT not only helps them minimize their emotional disturbance but also substitute their dysfunctional, self-defeating behaviour with useful, self-helping behaviour. That means that REBT aims at helping people feel better and also get better in the sense that they can cope with their problems effectively. It is not the goal of REBT to teach people just to liberate themselves from their emotional disturbances and to experience some sort of serenity.
2. **Second goal:** The aim of the REBT practitioner is to help his client totally restructure his personality so that he has minimum irrational beliefs and philosophies about himself, others and the

conditions he lives in. This kind of restructuring is expected to achieve another long-lasting result, namely, the client becomes less disturbable in the future. This is precisely the second goal of the REBT practitioner. He not only wants to reduce the client's disturbance, but reduce his disturbability.

3. **Third goal:** As the main causes of people's emotional disturbances and dysfunctional, self-defeating behaviours are rooted in their irrational beliefs or irrational philosophies about themselves, others and the world around them, REBT teaches them to get rid of those irrational philosophies and imbibe rational philosophies about themselves, others and the world they occupy. This is an important step in the direction of helping people feel better and get better. REBT then turns its attention to the third goal, namely, to encourage people to live happily and to engage in self-actualizing pursuits.

These goals of therapy are presented in somewhat idealistic terms. As the therapist himself does not believe in any musturbatory ideologies, about his therapeutic work, he does not insist on perfectly achieving those goals with respect to all his clients under all circumstances. He is ready to make compromises and help his clients feel and also get better as much as possible.

Analysis of Cases 5.1, 5.2 and 5.3 in Light of the Therapeutic Goals

Keeping these goals in mind, let us now see what help the REBT practitioner can offer to Aditi, Vikram and Saniya.

Aditi: An REBT practitioner's focus would be helping Aditi overcome her irrational philosophy that she *must* do perfectly well in the job interview. She then will be taught to accept the alternative rational philosophy that it will be very much desirable to do well in the job interview so that the probability of her getting the job increases. This new philosophy will largely replace her unhealthy emotion of anxiety by the healthy emotion of concern. This will induce her to give the job interview calmly and intelligently. Then it can be said that her therapist helped her to both, feel better and get better.

Vikram: How will the therapist help Vikram? He will teach him to overcome his irrational philosophy that others, and especially his boss, *must* be kind and just to him. He will be also encouraged to acquire the alternative rational philosophy that it will be good if others, and especially his boss, are kind and just to him, but there is no reason why they have to be so. This rational philosophy will replace his unhealthy emotion of anger at his boss by the healthy emotion of annoyance. This, in turn, will help him to behave with his boss, and even others, in a more tolerant and friendly manner. It can hence be said that his therapist helps him to feel better as well as get better.

Saniya: Finally, if Saniya approaches an REBT practitioner, she will learn to give up her irrational philosophy that conditions in the world *must* make things easy for her. This will also help her to assimilate the alternative rational philosophy that although it would be nice if all the conditions in the world are hassle-free, there is no reason why they *must* be so. Consequently, her unhealthy depression will slowly fade and she will feel the healthy emotion of frustration. Then, she will exert herself to implement the diet prescribed by her doctor. In short, she will not only feel better but also start getting better.

In reality, however, the client is rarely handicapped by only one musturbatory ideology and one unhealthy emotion. Usually, he is a victim of two or all the three musturbatory ideologies, although the proportion of musturbatory ideologies in the mind differs from client to client. Similarly, the client is rarely disturbed by only primary emotions such as anxiety, anger, depression, etc. Mostly, he tends to create secondary and even tertiary emotional disturbances in his mind. The REBT practitioner not only helps him to surrender his main musturbatory ideologies and all the vestiges of those ideologies in his mind but also his secondary and tertiary emotional disturbances.

Three Insights in REBT

REBT helps clients develop three insights in the therapeutic process. The insights gain in REBT differs from psychoanalytic insights. Unlike Psychoanalytic, REBT doesn't assume that acquisition of insights automatically lead to behavioural change. Insights in REBT refer to deep understanding of the concepts which provoke the person to go to the next level of the therapeutic process. The three insights are as follows:

Insight 1: The main cause of our emotional disturbance is not the activating event but it is our current irrational belief system. This insight creates the awareness that we largely create our own disturbance by making absolutistic demand from ourselves, others and life. This insight helps the person in taking charge of his own emotional disturbance.

Insight 2: No matter how we originally become disturbed, we feel upset today because we are still re-indoctrinating ourselves with the same kinds of irrational beliefs that we originated in the past. We acquire many irrational beliefs from our parents and from society in the childhood and cling to them because we keep repeating them to ourselves. Our self-conditioning is therefore important than our early conditioning (Ellis & MacLaren, 1998). This insight brings the awareness that past traumatic events could be the onset of our emotional disturbance, but we have a choice to reduce our emotional disturbance by not clinging to these irrational beliefs in the present.

Insight 3: If we need to reduce our emotional disturbance, we need to constantly work and practise in the present and in the future, to think, feel and act against irrational belief system. As we have biological, learned and habituated tendencies to maintain these beliefs, cognitive, emotive and behavioural work and practice is needed (Ellis & Whiteley, 1979). REBT believes that we do not change our irrational beliefs automatically after gaining the first two insights. If we want to bring about a long-term change in our self-defeating thoughts and behaviour, the only way is to work hard at changing the irrational beliefs.

REBT holds that we have a capacity to change how we think, feel and behave. However, we easily slip into absolutistic thinking as it is deeply rooted in our mind. When the client gets all three insights and works on them strongly and persistently, he reaches the elegant solution of getting better than merely feel better. This is the last juncture of therapeutic process where the client becomes self-empowered to pursue the rational philosophy of life and, if he backslides, he still can achieve his goal through lifelong work and practice on the insights.

References

DiGiuseppe, R. (1991). A rational-emotive model of assessment. In M.E. Bernard (Ed.), *Using Rational-Emotive Therapy Effectively*. New York, NY: Plenum.

Dryden, W. (1994). *Progress in Rational Emotive Behaviour Therapy*. London: Whurr.

Dryden, W., & Branch. (2008). *The Fundamentals of Rational Emotive Behaviour Therapy.* A Training Handbook (2nd ed., p. 37). West Sussex: John Wiley & Sons Ltd.

Ellis, A. (1967). In A.R. Mahrer (Ed.), *The Goals of Psychotherapy*. New York, NY: Appleton-Century-Crofts.

Ellis, A. (1972). In A. Ellis & C. MacLaren (Eds.), (2003). *Rational Emotive Behavior Therapy: A Therapist's Guide* (4th ed., p. 38). Impact Publishers.

———. (1977). *A Garland of Rational Songs.* New York, NY: Albert Ellis Institute.

———. (1979). Rejoinder: Elegant and inelegant RET. In A. Ellis & J.M. Whitley (Eds.), *Theoretical and Empirical Foundations of RET* (pp. 240–67). New York, NY: Brunner.

———. (1994). *Reason and Emotion in Psychotherapy: A Comprehensive Method of Treating Human Disturbances* (Revised and updated, pp. 221–24). New York, NY: Carol Publishing.

———. (1999). *Make Yourself Happy and Remarkably Less Disturbable* (p. 141). Mumbai: Jaico Publishing House.

———. (2001). *Feeling Better, Getting Better, Staying Better: Profound Self-Help for Your Emotions.* California: Impact Publishers, Inc.

Ellis, A., & Dryden, W. (1997). *The Practice of Rational Emotive Behavior Therapy* (2nd ed., p. 30). New York, NY: Springer Publishing Company.

Ellis, A., & MacLaren, C. (1998). The REBT theory of personality disturbance and change. *Rational-Emotive Behavior Therapy: A Therapist's Guide* (p. 38). Volume 2 of Practical therapist series. Atascadero, CA: Impact Publishers.

Ellis, A., & Whiteley, J. (1979). *Theoretical and Empirical Foundations of Rational-Emotive Therapy* (pp. 46–47). Brooks/Cole series in Counseling Psychology. California: Brooks/Cole Publishing Company.

Ellis, A., Gordon, J., Neenan, M., & Palmer, S. (2003). *Stress-Counseling: A Rational Emotive Behavioral Approach* (p. 41). Continuum, NY: SAGE.

Ellis, A., Young, J., & Lockwood, G. (1987). Cognitive therapy and rational-emotive therapy: A dialog. *Journal of Cognitive Psychotherapy: An International Quarterly, 1*(4), 205–55.

Grieger, R., & Boyd, J. (1980). *Rational-Emotive Therapy: A Skills-Based Approach.* New York, NY: Van Nostrand Reinhold.

Phadke, K.M., & Khear, R. (1998). *Counselling in Industry: Rational Approach* (1st ed., p. 115). Mumbai: Himalaya Publishing House.

Rogers, C. (1942). *Counseling and Psychotherapy: Newer Concepts in Practice.* Cambridge, MA: Houghton Mifflin.

Walen, S., DiGiuseppe, R., & Wessler, R. (1980). *A Practitioner's Guide to Rational-Emotive-Therapy* (pp. 32, 164). New York, NY: Oxford University Press.

Further Readings

Ellis, A. (1980). Rational-emotive therapy and cognitive behavior therapy: Similarities and differences. *Cognitive Therapy and Research, 4*(4), 325–40.

———. (1996). *Better, Deeper, and More Enduring Brief Therapy.* New York, NY: Brunner/Mazel.

Ellis, A., & MacLaren, C. (1998). *Rational Emotive Behavior Therapy: A Therapist's Guide.* San Luis Obispo, CA: Impact Publishers.

9

Therapeutic Techniques of REBT

After understanding the therapeutic process of REBT in detail, it is the time to review its therapeutic techniques. In this chapter, we shall address the problem: How does the therapist actually use REBT to help the client overcome his emotional disturbance? In order to understand the current methodology of REBT, it would be worthwhile to review Ellis' original therapeutic technique when REBT was just a newborn baby.

Original therapeutic techniques: Let us recall that when Ellis presented the paper, 'Rational Psychotherapy' at the Annual Convention of the APA in 1956, he hoisted a flag of rebellion. What were the main targets of his rebellion? His major quarrel was with the technique of delving into the childhood experiences of the client and the technique of remaining passive while doing therapy. The first technique was largely a product of the Freudian psychoanalysis, whereas the second technique was mainly a manifestation of Carl Rogers' widespread influence on psychotherapists.

When Ellis started his private practice, he did not bother to go into the childhood experiences of the clients. Believing that their psychological disturbances were caused by their currently held irrational beliefs, he actively and directly challenged, questioned, examined and disputed the irrational beliefs underlying their disturbances and then taught them alternative rational beliefs. If the learned professional psychologists who heard his presentation of these cases were shocked, it was quite understandable. After all, Ellis had shaken the very foundation of the prevailing concepts of psychotherapy.

Naturally, Ellis met with resistance and even opposition from a large number of the well-established psychotherapists. Their chief objection was that REBT was too cognitive and oblivious of the affective or emotive aspect of man's psychological disturbance. This objection was not totally wrong as Ellis' technique of disputing the irrational beliefs of the client was certainly focusing on cognitive, ideational or philosophic aspect of man's psychological disturbance. However, it was emotive too in the sense that the process of disputation was definitely forceful and energetic. On the whole, it cannot be denied that in the original version of REBT, the therapist's main thrust was on challenging and changing the client's disturbance creating cognitions.

Ellis admitted that in the early days of REBT, he concentrated on challenging and changing the client's irrational beliefs and helping him acquire alternative rational beliefs. This kind of change in the client's philosophy of life was helping him reduce his emotional disturbance and then go about solving his practical problems.

We can imagine how Ellis would have helped Aditi, Vikram and Saniya, (Cases 5.1, 5.2 and 5.3) had they approached him when REBT was in its nascent form. He would have directly, actively and forcefully disputed their musturbatory ideologies and urged them to assimilate alternative rational beliefs so that they would reduce their anxiety, anger and depression respectively. Then armed with newly learned rational beliefs or philosophies of life, they might have harnessed their mental resources to tackle their individual practical problem. Ellis would have worked at changing their faulty cognitions, disturbing emotions and dysfunctional behaviour. Surely, he would have disputed their irrational beliefs quite forcefully and energetically. This technique would have helped those three cases, as it was helping many other clients.

The original version of REBT, though more efficient and effective than many other contemporary therapies, was overemphasizing man's cognitions or philosophies of life. As a matter of fact, the thinking or cognitive process is just one of the three mental processes of man. The other two are feeling or emoting and doing or behaving. Therefore, Ellis was taken to task by his critics for neglecting the emotive and behavioural processes of man's mental life.

The criticism was not completely justifiable because when Ellis disputed the client's irrational beliefs, he was not passive, cold and dry. On the contrary, he disputed the client's beliefs in a lively, emotive and forceful way. When he used to practise as a marriage and family counsellor as well as a sex therapist before he invented RT, he used to give behavioural assignments to the client. He was never focusing only on the thinking or cognitive process of man. However, the name of his newly invented system of psychotherapy, namely, RT, did give the impression that his therapeutic technique was exclusively concentrating on man's cognitive process.

Yet Ellis confessed that he made a great mistake when he called his system of psychotherapy RT because many people have some aversion to the word 'rational'. We have seen in Chapter 7 how the word 'rational' is commonly perceived synonymous to the terms 'logical, scientific, cold or unemotional', although, by the word 'rational' Ellis meant 'sensible, reasonable and practical'. Ellis thought it would have been better if he had called his system cognitive, cognitive-behavioural or cognitive-emotive-behavioural therapy in the first place.

In fairness to Ellis, it is necessary to point out that even in the very first formal presentation of rational therapy, he had emphasized the interactive, interdependent and holistic nature of the cognitive, emotive and behavioural processes of man. He never said or believed that these three processes are disparate.

There is no doubt that Epictetus's view that cognition is the basis of emotion is the cornerstone of REBT. Challenging and disputing the client's irrational beliefs can be largely done on the cognitive or intellectual level. Generally, this technique gives good results. In order to get better results, disputing the client's irrational beliefs had better be done on an emotional as well as a behavioural level. This three-pronged attack on the client's irrational beliefs is often more effective in bringing about more thoroughgoing and long-lasting changes in the client's personality.

Three types of therapeutic techniques: When an REBT therapist deals with the clients, he takes into consideration a number of background factors such as his age, gender, education, ability to grasp, personality traits, socio-economic factors, etc. to finalize the structure of therapeutic process. If required, he changes it during the process. The time required for the completion of the entire therapeutic process differs from person to person. However, one can definitely say that REBT takes lesser time than other therapies such as psychoanalysis, which are both time-consuming and expensive.

REBT is highly eclectic, and it adapts a multimodal approach. It consists of a variety of therapeutic techniques, some of which are borrowed from other psychotherapeutic systems. Ellis welcomed any technique if it can achieve goals that are in agreement with the REBT theory. This eclecticism of REBT is appropriately called 'theoretically consistent eclecticism' by Dr Windy Dryden (1986). This means REBT uses almost any technique if it can be adapted to the purpose of detecting and disputing the client's irrational beliefs so that they can be replaced by alternative rational beliefs.

For the sake of convenience, the techniques used in REBT can be classified under three heads—cognitive, emotive and behavioural.

However, it is necessary to bear in mind that almost all the techniques include cognitive, emotive and behavioural components as these components are not independent of each other.

1. **Cognitive:** These techniques are used to modify cognitive or thought process. In common language, we can say that they appeal to the 'head' part of the clients.
2. **Emotive:** These techniques are used to bring changes in unhealthy emotions. In common language, we can say that they harness the power of 'heart' of the clients.
3. **Behavioural:** These techniques are used to bring changes in dysfunctional behaviour. In common language, we can say that they emphasize 'muscles' or 'hand' part of the clients.

An REBT therapist launches a crusade against the irrational beliefs in the mind of the clients by using head, heart and muscles. Although a large number of techniques are used in REBT under each head, we are now going to discuss the most salient among them. We will also see how these techniques will help our three cases, Aditi (Case 5.1), Vikram (Case 5.2) and Saniya (Case 5.3). In order to explain cognitive techniques, we will take Aditi's case (Case 5.1). Emotive techniques will be explained with the help of Vikram's case (Case 5.2) and behavioural techniques will be seen in light of Saniya's case (Case 5.3).

Cognitive Techniques

Cognitive Disputation

From the very beginning, the process of disputing (D) has remained the most commonly used cognitive technique in REBT. The technique consists of arguing with the client so as to help him give up his irrational beliefs and internalize alternative rational beliefs instead. Irrational beliefs of the clients are challenged by the didactic or Socratic style. A didactic style involves a therapist's explanation of different terms referring to rational and irrational beliefs. The Socratic style refers to identify and dispute irrational beliefs. Radical questions are asked to the clients to present the evidence for holding these beliefs. In cognitive disputation, the therapist aims at changing the contents of his thoughts that create his emotional disturbance and intensively challenges the client's deep-rooted musturbatory ideologies.

REBT is so well known for its technique of disputing the client's irrational beliefs that some commentators on REBT conclude that REBT means disputation! Of course, this is an overgeneralization. The truth is that disputation occupies the central place among all techniques of REBT so much so, that REBT minus the technique of disputation is no REBT at all! In 1955, Ellis introduced the technique of openly disputing and changing cognitions to modern psychotherapy. Afterwards, various forms of cognitive behaviour therapy followed REBT's footsteps with or without giving credit to Ellis for this valuable addition to therapist's armamentarium.

According to Ellis, disputation is the most elegant of all the techniques used in REBT. He even goes to the extent of saying that disputation is 'probably the most elegant of all the prevailing psychotherapeutic techniques that have ever been invented'.

Socratic dialogues: However, Ellis does not claim that he invented this technique. On the contrary, he admitted that philosophers down the ages, starting from Socrates, have been using this technique. We may go even further and say that although Socrates spent his life in disputing conventional beliefs of the young and teaching philosophy to them, he was not the inventor of the technique of disputation. It was methodically practised by Zeno who was a disciple of Parmenides, but Socrates practised and developed it. Similarly, among the currently prevailing psychotherapies, REBT has certainly specialized in this time-honoured technique.

Unfortunately, REBT's emphasis on arguing with the client has been misunderstood by some critics. They wrongly conclude that REBT is equal to shaming argumentative therapy in which the therapist struggles to prove his intellectual superiority and expose the intellectual bankruptcy of the client. In reality, the therapist behaves with the client in a very humane manner and aims at helping him overcome his unhealthy emotions and modify his handicapping behaviour. Certainly, it is not his goal to belittle the client by parading his intellectual superiority.

ABC theory: In view of his goal of helping the client get rid of his unhealthy emotions, the therapist endeavours to show him that his unhealthy emotions stem from his irrational cognitions. In other words, he helps the client appreciate that his unhealthy emotions are not directly caused by some events in his life. Rather, they are caused by faulty evaluations of some events in his life. Once the client understands the

B–C connection in the A × B = C theory of emotional disturbance, the therapist asks him whether a change in his irrational beliefs is required for bringing about a change in his unhealthy emotions. Only when the client admits that he had better learn to give up his irrational beliefs, the therapist begins to dispute those beliefs and proceeds to teach him how he can dispute those beliefs on his own. On the contrary, if the therapist begins to challenge or dispute the client's irrational beliefs without his consent, he can hardly be considered an REBT practitioner.

We are now ready to learn how the therapist actually uses the technique of disputing the beliefs of clients. Surely, the therapist first explains to the client the A × B = C theory of emotional disturbance. He then ensures that the client admits that he is mainly responsible for his emotional disturbance and that in order to get rid of his emotional disturbance, he had better change his faulty thinking.

'D' step: How does the therapist move on to dispute (D) the client's beliefs? A careful observation of this process reveals its complexity. Phadke (1968–2003) corresponded with Ellis on 23 December 1975 to point out that the process of disputation can be logically broken down into three steps. The first step consists of detecting the client's faulty beliefs. How can the therapist dispute the client's beliefs unless first he clearly identifies those beliefs? The second step, of course, consists of actually disputing or challenging the client's beliefs detected in the first step. The third step consists of discriminating between the rational and irrational beliefs of the clients.

So the three-fold components of step D are as follows:

- Detection (detecting the beliefs)
- Debating (debating or disputing those beliefs)
- Discriminating (discriminating between the rational and irrational parts of those beliefs)

It is a tribute to Ellis' open-mindedness and magnanimity that not only did he agree with Phadke's suggestion but also generously acknowledged his humble contribution to the theory and the practice of REBT in many of his subsequent articles and books (Ellis, 1977).

Analysis of Case 5.1 in Light of Cognitive Techniques

Aditi and Ellis: Just imagine that Aditi has approached Ellis to seek his help to reduce her job-anxiety. In order to understand how Ellis used the technique of disputation while working with his client, let us see how he might offer therapy to Aditi. After listening to her problem, Ellis will ask her what outcome she expects from the therapy. Thus, first of all, Ellis will help her fix the goal (G) of therapy. They will then decide that the goal is to make her get rid of her unhealthy emotion of anxiety and face the interview for which she has received a call. This two-fold goal is well within the purview of REBT.

B–C connection: Ellis will then teach Aditi that her anxiety is not caused by the call to attend the interview but by her interpretation and evaluation of the prospect of giving the interview. In order to teach this to Aditi, Ellis may ask her how a hundred girls will feel if they receive similar call for the job interview. Ellis follows this method of probing with a view to help her realize that different girls will feel different emotions besides anxiety. In this way, Ellis will show her how different human beings react to the same situation according to their beliefs about that situation. He will teach her to shoulder the responsibility of her anxiety and the resulting avoidance of facing the job interview.

When Aditi clearly sees that her own belief is largely responsible for her emotional and behavioural problem, Ellis will ask her whether she considers it necessary to change her belief for solving her emotional and behavioural problem. Only when she understands the relevance of the B–C connection in the A × B = C theory, vis-à-vis her problem, she will agree to work at changing her belief.

Detection of the belief: Ellis is now set to use the technique of disputing Aditi's belief. The first step in the process of disputation is to detect the belief underlying Aditi's emotional disturbance, namely, anxiety. As per the REBT theory of emotional disturbance, Ellis follows the general rule: detect the '*must*' explicit or implicit in the client's mind. He will ask Aditi what she talks to herself about the interview when she experiences anxiety or what thoughts go on in her mind when she feels anxious about facing the interview. Normally, with a little probing, he will detect that what she tells herself about the job interview is some variation of Musturbatory Ideology 1 and is something like, 'I absolutely *must* do perfectly well in any interview and *must* be approved by people I consider significant or else I am an *inadequate and unlovable person*'.

Derivatives of the belief: When Ellis persists in his efforts to detect other ideas underlying Aditi's anxiety, he will come across three major ideas that are actually the derivatives of this musturbatory ideology. They can be thus summarized as follows:

1. It is awful, meaning more than 100 per cent bad, if my ignorance is exposed and if I am disapproved by the people I consider significant in my life.
2. I cannot have any happiness in my life if my ignorance is exposed.
3. If my ignorance is exposed, it will mean that I am a worthless, subhuman person who deserves nothing good in life.

The second step in the process of disputation is to challenge Aditi's musturbatory ideology and its derivatives. It requires a process of arguing with Aditi with objective to reveal the irrationality of her musturbatory ideology and its derivatives. Of course, in order to argue with Aditi, Ellis needs to have some criteria of rationality.

It may be recalled from Chapter 5 (Table 5.1) that Dr Maxie C. Maultsby, Jr, propounded five criteria of rational thinking which were accepted by Ellis. Ellis, as well as other practitioners of REBT, had been using those criteria of rationality as guidelines for disputing the beliefs of their clients. Subsequently, Ellis revised those criteria and formulated only three criteria of rational thinking. Since then, he had been teaching his clients to assess whether their beliefs are rational or irrational in the light of those simplified criteria. Let us review those rules of rational thinking in order to understand how Ellis will dispute Aditi's beliefs.

1. **Functional:** Does it help the client over the long run to believe this? If it hinders him, what thought would help him reach his goals better and feel better?
2. **Factual:** Is the client's belief/thinking consistent with facts? If it isn't, what is?
3. **Logical:** Is the client's belief/thinking logical? If not, what would make more sense logically?

Armed with these three criteria of rationality, Ellis will meticulously and rigorously challenge all the ideas that create and keep up Aditi's anxiety which he has detected in the first step of disputation. When Ellis successfully executes the second step, he will almost simultaneously complete the third step in the process of disputation, namely, to teach the client to discriminate between the rational and irrational components of his philosophy of life. A sample of the therapy he would offer to Aditi is given below.

Aditi: I have to get the job for which I have applied; and who will offer it to me if I don't succeed in the interview?

Ellis: What do you exactly mean when you say that you have to get the job for which you have applied?

Aditi: I mean that I *must* get that job and therefore *must* do very well in the interview.

Ellis: Do you think that those thoughts in your mind are likely to help you achieve your goal of succeeding in the interview?

Aditi: They may or may not. But I became very anxious with those thoughts in my mind.

Ellis: Is that anxiety likely to help you do well in the interview?

Aditi: No, on the contrary, it is likely to hinder my performance in the interview. That is why I feel like avoiding the ordeal of the interview.

Ellis: Good! So do you understand how your own thinking makes it difficult for you to achieve your aim?

Aditi: Yes, but what can I do to overcome those anxiety creating thoughts in my mind?

Ellis: One thing that you can do is to think of some alternative thoughts that may be useful to you in achieving your objective. Can you find some other thoughts that may meet your requirements?

Aditi: I think it would be better if I tell myself that I definitely want the job for which I have applied. It is very much desirable that I focus on doing quite well in the interview.

Ellis: Which emotion will be created in your mind by those alternative thoughts? Can you make a guess?

Aditi: I think those alternative thoughts will make me feel concerned about the interview. They will motivate me to accept the challenge of facing the so-called ordeal of interview.

(The dialogues show how Ellis challenges Aditi's ideas by using the first of the three criteria of rational thinking [functional] and thereby follows the first step in the process of disputation. Briefly, the criterion states that rational thinking takes a man towards his goal.)

Ellis: Good! Now are you able to see the difference in the thoughts that create anxiety about the interview and the thoughts that create concern about the interview in your mind?

Aditi: Definitely! I can easily see that the thoughts that create anxiety in my mind are obviously irrational because they tend to interfere with my goal attainment.

Ellis: What can you say about thoughts that are likely to create a feeling of concern in your mind?

Aditi: Those thoughts are obviously rational or sensible.

Ellis: Because?

Aditi: Because they help me remain focused on my objective without becoming anxious.

Ellis: All right.

> (*This dialogue shows how Ellis helps Aditi discriminate between the rational and irrational thoughts by using the first of the three criteria of rational thinking and thereby follows the third step in the process of disputation. As you know, the first criterion states that rational thinking takes a man towards his goal.*)

Aditi: I have also clearly understood the difference between unhealthy and healthy emotions which you taught me when you explained your A × B = C theory of emotional disturbance.

Ellis: I am glad to hear that you have now understood the difference between healthy and unhealthy emotions. Can you elaborate what you have understood?

Aditi: I can clearly see that anxiety is an unhealthy emotion because it keeps me disturbed and also urges me to avoid the interview. Whereas, concern is quite a healthy emotion because it motivates me to accept the challenge of facing the interview and helps me focus on how to do well in the interview.

Ellis: Yes, but you can get rid of your handicapping anxiety by telling yourself some other sentences also.

Aditi: For example?

Ellis: You can tell yourself something like, 'I don't give a hoot whether I get the job or not for which I have applied'.

Aditi: I think ... if I tell myself these kinds of sentences, I will get rid of my anxiety and concern too! But such sentences will give a deathblow to my goal. So they are also to be considered irrational.

Ellis: Good! You have certainly understood the A × B = C theory of emotional disturbance and the first criteria of distinguishing between rational thinking and irrational thinking.

Aditi: I am glad that you are satisfied with my progress.

Ellis: Yes, your progress is commendable. However, let us briefly see whether you can examine the other sentences which are responsible for creating and maintaining anxiety in your mind. You have already identified those sentences. Do you remember those sentences?

Aditi: Yes, those sentences are 'It will be terrible if I perform miserably in the interview and consequently don't get the job I have applied for. I will then not be able to show my face to significant people in my life. It will be impossible for me to stand that situation. Moreover, my failure to do well in the interview and get the job will prove that I am a worthless person who deserves to be totally condemned'.

Ellis: Yes, you have correctly recalled the sentences responsible for your anxiety and desire to avoid facing the interview. Do you think that those sentences are rational?

Aditi: No! On the contrary, they are to be considered irrational because they make me feel anxious. That anxiety interferes with my efforts to focus on doing well in the interview.

Ellis: All right! Can you think of some alternative sentences that may help you achieve your goal?

Aditi: Yes, I can tell myself something like, 'It will be disappointing and disadvantageous if I don't do well in the interview and then fail to get the job. But it will not be terrible. I don't see any reason why I shall not be able to show my face to significant people in my life in case I don't get the job I want. I can definitely stand that situation. Moreover, my failure to get the job will only mean that I shall have to continue my efforts to get a suitable job. I shall learn something from my failure without condemning myself or becoming upset even if some people condemn me for my failure'.

Ellis: These alternative sentences are ...

Aditi: These alternative sentences are rational because they will create the healthy emotion of concern instead of the unhealthy emotion of anxiety in my mind. The emotion of concern, in turn, will help me focus on doing well in the interview so that I may get the job I want.

(Ellis ensures that Aditi has clearly understood the technique of disputation by asking her to dispute the remaining sentences which are responsible for creating anxiety in her mind. It is obvious that Aditi has understood how to use the first criterion of rational thinking.)

Ellis: Very good! Now we are ready to learn the second criterion of rationality and to challenge all the sentences which create anxiety in your mind as well as an impulse to avoid the interview. Do you remember the second criterion of rational thinking?

Aditi: Yes. The second criterion is 'Is my thinking consistent with facts? If it isn't, what is?'

Ellis: You are right. Let us go back to the first among all the ideas which create anxiety in your mind. Can you recall that idea?

Aditi: Yes. My first thought is 'I *must* get the job for which I have applied'.

Ellis: How will you dispute this idea in the light of second criterion of rationality?

Aditi: Can you help me in forming the questions?

Ellis: Certainly! Here are few questions—Where is the evidence to say that I *must*? Where has it been written that I *must* get what I want? Is there any universal law which compels me to get this job? Do I have a control on all the conditions of getting this job? On what basis am I making this compulsion on myself?

Aditi: Yes, I realize that I cannot prove any evidence to hold this idea in my mind. It is an absolutistic demand of my mind which has no factual base. Obviously, this is an irrational idea because this is inconsistent with reality. The reality is that I can and often do fail to get what I demand.

Ellis: It is now necessary to go through the remaining ideas which create anxiety in your mind and challenge them by using the second criterion of rational thinking.

Aditi: It is not necessary to do so. I can easily see that those ideas are also not consistent with facts.

Ellis: You are right. But let us just consider one among those ideas.

Aditi: Which one?

Ellis: When you feel anxious, you are telling yourself, 'It will be *terrible* if I perform miserably in the interview and consequently don't get the job I have applied for'.

Aditi: Why do you want me to focus on this particular idea?

Ellis: Can you guess why I have picked up this idea?

Aditi: Yes, I think it is difficult to check whether this idea is consistent with facts because I am not sure what I mean by the word *terrible*.

Ellis: Very good! What do you propose to do before you challenge that idea in light of the second criterion of rational thinking?

Aditi: First, I had better state that idea in such a way that I can check whether it is consistent with reality. For example, 'If I perform miserably in the interview and consequently fail to get the job, then I will incur such and such losses'.

Ellis: Okay! What is the advantage of clearly stating your meaning of the word *terrible*?

Aditi: It will help me check whether my idea is consistent with facts. (*Ellis is emphasizing the importance of being precise about expressing our ideas. Many times imprecisely formulated sentences create confusion in the client's mind. Besides, imprecise ideas are difficult to check with facts.*)

Ellis: How will you dispute this idea?

Aditi: I will ask questions to myself, such as, what do I mean by *terrible*? Is it terrible or am I making it *terrible*? Why is it *terrible* when life doesn't give me what it *must* give me? Will it be unpleasant or terrible? If I don't get this job, what *terrible* will happen exactly? Will I faint or be hospitalized immediately?

Ellis: (*Laughingly*) Now I am sure you will examine the remaining ideas underlying your anxiety quite successfully. What will you do afterwards?

Aditi: I will formulate alternative rational ideas which will be consistent with facts so that they will create the feeling of concern in my mind and also help me focus on doing well in the interview.

Ellis: Fine! May we move on to the third criterion of rationality?

Aditi: Yes, the third criterion of rational thinking is 'Is my thinking logical? If not, what would make more sense logically?'

Ellis: That's right! Let us go back to the first among all your ideas which create anxiety in your mind. Can you recall that idea?

Aditi: Yes. My first thought is 'I *must* get the job for which I have applied'.

Ellis: Can you challenge this thought in the light of the third criterion of rationality?

Aditi: This is an irrational thought. The conclusion that I *have to* get the job applied for does not logically follow from the statement that I strongly want to get the job for which I have applied.

Ellis: Can you tell me why your conclusion is illogical?

Aditi: My conclusion is illogical because my or anybody's desire, no matter how intense, to get something is not a sufficient condition for the fulfilment of that desire. I will ask questions to myself, such as, will it be logical if I equate desire to fulfilment? Will anybody's desire sufficient condition for its fulfilment?

Ellis: All right! What will you do now?

Aditi: I will challenge all the remaining ideas which give rise to anxiety in my mind by using the third criterion of rational thinking.

Ellis: I am sure you will be able to challenge those ideas correctly. Let us see how you challenge just one among those ideas.

Aditi: Which one?

Ellis: That idea is 'My failure to do well in the interview and get the job will prove that I am a *worthless* person who deserves to be totally condemned'.

Aditi: Oh, this idea is non-sensible! Even if I fail to do well in the interview and get the job, how will I prove logically that I am a worthless person who deserves to be totally condemned?

Ellis: Can you tell me why this particular anxiety creating idea is illogical?

Aditi: This idea represents an exaggerated conclusion. My failure will not warrant any evaluation about my total personality.

Ellis: What can be logically concluded from your failures?

Aditi: One logical conclusion can be that if I do not get the job, I will have a setback. However, it does not prove that I am a worthless person who deserves to be condemned. In fact, it is a far-fetched conclusion that if a human being fails in any undertaking, his entire personality deserves to be condemned.

Ellis: Good! Let us suppose that you do very well in the interview and get the job. Then will it be logical to say that you are a great person who deserves universal praise and some huge rewards?

Aditi: This conclusion also contains an overgeneralization. If I am successful in the interview and get the job, it does not mean I am a totally successful or a great person. It only means I shall have some advantages. It is better to draw conclusions about advantages and disadvantages of getting and not getting this job. It is illogical to draw any conclusion about my total personality on the basis of my success or failure in getting the job.

(Ellis is spending quite some time in checking whether Aditi has understood the difference in man's performance and his totality or his very being. In REBT, this distinction is the basis of teaching people how to accept themselves and others unconditionally.)

Ellis: There is no doubt that you have clearly understood how to use the third criterion of rational thinking. What do you propose to do now?

Aditi: Of course, I will challenge the remaining ideas which create the unhealthy emotion of anxiety in my mind.

Ellis: Good! What is the next thing to be done?

Aditi: I then have to formulate alternative logical ideas which will create a feeling of concern in my mind and also help me focus on doing well in the interview.

Hopefully, the excerpts of dialogues between Aditi and Ellis serve the purpose of understanding the nature of disputation as a technique of therapy. However, there is nothing sacrosanct about this method of disputing the client's irrational beliefs. Almost any dialogue that teaches or persuades the client to surrender his irrational beliefs and learn rational beliefs can be considered effective disputation. Box 9.1 presents the examples of questions that can be used for disputation.

Box 9.1

Some Suggestions on Disputation Questions

1. Where is the evidence to support the existence of this belief?
2. Where is the proof?
3. Is it consistent with reality?
4. Is it true?
5. Why is that so?
6. Is it not an overgeneralization? Why?
7. Is it not an exaggeration? Why?
8. Can I prove it?
9. Why it *must* be?
10. On what basis did I agree with this idea?
11. What do the data/the facts show?
12. Why does it have to be so?
13. Is this belief logical?
14. Does it logically follow from my rational belief?
15. Where is holding this belief getting me?
16. Is it helpful?
17. Why would I be destroyed if I don't …?
18. Let's assume the worst. I am doing the very worst thing. Now why *must* I not do it?
19. How would that be so terrible?
20. What good things can happen if … happens?
21. Explain why I can't stand it?
22. Can't I be happy even if I don't get what you want?
23. Why *must* I/others/life not?
24. Where is the evidence?
25. Is that true? Why not?

Cognitive Homework

This technique aligns well with the third insight of REBT, that is, work! work! practice! This assignment is used to help the client practice the technique of disputing his irrational beliefs in the time outside therapy sessions. The client could be feeling and behaving according to his irrational beliefs for years. Therefore, it is necessary that he regularly spends some time in detecting and disputing his irrational beliefs. To facilitate the practice of his newly acquired skill of disputing irrational beliefs, Ellis and his associates have designed a number of homework sheets. Those homework sheets offer the client a structured method of practising the technique of disputing his irrational beliefs.[2]

In Aditi's case, Ellis will give her a homework sheet and ask her to complete it as a cognitive homework assignment outside therapy sessions. She will be asked to identify adversities (A) during the time outside the session and try to dispute irrational beliefs with help of the insights received in the session. She will attempt to do this homework in light of what she continues to learn in therapy sessions. Ellis will then check her homework and provide some constructive feedback to her. In this way, he will help her strengthen her learning and consolidate the gains derived from therapy sessions.

Proselytizing

In this technique, the clients are asked to help others in solving their problems. If it is someone else's problem, the client can view it more objectively than his own problem. The therapist encourages the client to use REBT to help his relatives, friends, acquaintances, etc., if they are willing to receive help for solving their emotional problems.

In Aditi's case, Ellis will ask her to offer help to some willing 'clients'. In the process of helping others, she will identify and dispute even her own irrational beliefs without herself feeling threatened. Thus, she will understand the main principles of REBT and learn how to use them to solve her own problems more confidently.

---

[2] Sample homework sheets for practice and solved are provided in Appendices I & II.

Recording Therapy Sessions

Recording therapy sessions is a great aid to the client as he can listen to the recordings whenever he needs and strengthens his learnings. After all, clients find it very difficult to recall everything that happens even in one therapy session. However, if their sessions are tape-recorded, they will listen to their own therapy sessions repeatedly and get more benefit. In Aditi's case, Ellis will tape-record his sessions with her and ask her to listen to them between sessions. If Aditi listens to the taped sessions with Ellis, she will pick up some aspects of therapy more clearly. Besides, Aditi may listen to these sessions as if she is listening to some other person's problem. This will enable her to be more objective about what is going on in therapy sessions. She may then derive more benefit from her therapy sessions.

Modelling

This is another technique designed to help the client look at his problem objectively. In this technique, the client is asked to choose any role model whom he admires and would like to emulate. This role model will provide a reference to the client in the path of problem solving. For example, Ellis can ask Aditi to think of somebody she knows or somebody she may have read or heard about and who can be considered as a model worth copying. Then he will ask her to visualize how that man will feel or behave even if he fails to do well in the job interview and as a result, does not get the job he wants.

Aditi's task is to note the differences between her thinking about the job interview until she learns to replace her irrational thoughts with more rational thoughts.

Bibliotherapy

In order to supplement therapy sessions, the therapist recommends the client to read articles, books, hear audiotapes, see videos, etc. It serves the purpose of reinforcing and consolidating his newly acquired rational beliefs. For example, Ellis may give Aditi some reading assignments with a view to supplementing his efforts to teach her how to think rationally about her problem. He will recommend Aditi the following two books which will strengthen her rational thinking: First, *How to Control Your Anxiety Before It Controls You* (Ellis, 2000), and the second, A *Guide to Rational Living* (Ellis & Harper, 1997).

Referenting

In simple terminology, it is a cost-benefit analysis. If Ellis wants to use this technique for Aditi, he will ask her to make a comprehensive list of the advantages of working at therapy and disadvantages of resisting it. She will be encouraged to keep this list readily available to her and read it 5–10 times a day. This technique will strengthen Aditi's efforts to work harder at therapy.

Emotive Techniques

The main purpose of all cognitive techniques is to detect, critically examine and replace the client's irrational philosophy of life. According to the A × B = C theory of emotional disturbance, if the client adopts a rational philosophy of life, he will derive lasting emotional and behavioural benefits. Keeping in mind this vital point, let us turn our attention to some emotive techniques frequently used in REBT.

Analysis of Case 5.2 in Light of Emotive Techniques

Vikram and Ellis: A simple way to understand emotive techniques is to turn our attention to Vikram—the second of our three cases. Imagine that Vikram has approached Ellis to seek help to overcome his anger and the resulting behavioural problem. How will Ellis use emotive techniques to help him?

Before we answer this question, it is necessary to bear in mind that at first, Ellis will dispute the irrational belief to which he is strongly adhering. That belief is Musturbatory Ideology 2, that is, 'other people absolutely *must* under all conditions treat me fairly and justly or else they are *rotten, damnable* people'. Ellis will dispute and demolish this irrational philosophy of life rooted in Vikram's mind and replace it with a more rational philosophy which may be stated as 'I would like other people to treat me fairly and justly. But there is no reason why they *must* do so. Even if they behave in unfair and unjust ways with me, they do not become rotten, damnable persons although their behaviour may be wrong or even immoral'.

Ellis will begin to use emotive techniques with a view to consolidating and strengthening Vikram's newly acquired rational philosophy of life, only after completing the first one. We now turn our attention to understand how Ellis will achieve this goal by using emotive techniques. We presume that he has already successfully disputed Vikram's irrational philosophy of life and replaced it with an alternative rational philosophy of life.

Unconditional Acceptance by Therapist

Whenever possible, an REBT practitioner endeavours to behave with the client in such a way that he feels like emulating his healthy philosophy of life. A method of doing so is to give the client unconditional acceptance irrespective of his bad or self-harming actions.

Therefore, Ellis will accept Vikram unconditionally in therapy sessions. He may think that some of Vikram's ways of dealing with his boss are not appropriate and he may bring this fact to Vikram's attention. Yet he will refrain from condemning Vikram for his improper behaviour. Nevertheless, he will ensure that Vikram will not condemn himself for his inappropriate ways of dealing with boss. In short, he will help Vikram review and rate his behaviour without rating himself or his totality.

Teaching USA and UOA

Ellis not only offers unconditional acceptance to Vikram but also teaches him what the concepts of USA and UOA mean and how to behave according to those concepts.

Ellis will teach him that a man's total personality, being too complex, cannot be adequately described by fixing a global descriptive label on his forehead. He will then help Vikram accept himself with his anger and his own self-defeating reaction to his boss and try to overcome those two handicaps without condemning himself. Further, Ellis will teach him to accept his boss unconditionally as a fallible human being without necessarily liking all his behaviour and traits.

Finally, Ellis will help him differentiate between the unhealthy emotion of anger and the healthy emotion of annoyance. When Vikram understands this difference, he will continue to feel annoyance at some of his boss' behaviour. This may motivate him to find out ways of coping with his boss' behaviour. However, he will not feel angry with his boss for his real or imagined unfair and unkind behaviour. Thus, he will learn to condemn the behaviour of a man without condemning the man himself, that is, his very being or totality. The excerpt of their dialogue would be as follows:

Ellis: Let's assume that your boss has ordered you to do some work in a dictatorial manner. You can still accept him unconditionally. Have you understood this?

Vikram: Yes, to a certain extent. However, it is still difficult for me to accept my boss when he does this discourteous act. If he is bad mannered, how can one still accept him unconditionally? Doesn't it mean that we give consent to his bad-mannered behaviour?

Ellis: Yes, it is difficult, but not impossible. Still you can accept him.

Vikram: How?

Ellis: First, tell me the definition of a 'bad person'.

Vikram: A person who creates harm to other people or behaves indecently with other people and does not have concern for the other people is a bad person.

Ellis: Suppose I meet a person who creates harm to the other people, behaves indecently with other people or does not have concern for the other people, which correct phrase *should* I use? Is he behaving badly or he is a 'bad person'.

Vikram: I got your point. Calling him a 'bad person' is an exaggeration.

Ellis: Why?

Vikram: Because it is not only wrong factually but logically inconsistent as well. Calling him a 'bad person' conveys the idea that he has always acted badly, is acting entirely badly and will continue to act badly until his death.

Ellis: Correct! Have you ever come across any such person?

Vikram: Certainly not!

Ellis: Do you think any such human being could have ever existed on this planet?

Vikram: I don't.

Ellis:	I am convinced that you have grasped the reason why it was wrong to dub your boss a 'bad person'. If you make a difference in 'behaving badly' and 'a bad person', what will be the consequence?
Vikram:	If I say that he is behaving badly, I accept that his bad behaviour is a part of his whole personality. There might be some good traits along with the bad ones. He is a mixture of both. When I labelled him 'bad', it did not help me functionally too.
Ellis:	How?
Vikram:	When I thought that he was a 'bad person', I angered myself too much and that, in turn, prevented me from undertaking some constructive action to solve the problem.
Ellis:	If you realize that, then ...
Vikram:	I will throw away that label, and all similar labels, like, 'nasty', 'crazy guy', 'bitch' and what not.
Ellis:	What would be the consequence of that?
Vikram:	It will be easy for me to accept them unconditionally.

(*Ellis is highlighting a very significant point of unconditional acceptance that even if you strongly dislike other's behaviour, you can still accept him with his good and bad behaviour and refrain from rating him globally as a person.*)

Rational Emotive Imagery

Many writers of self-help books, devotees of positive thinking such as Norman Vincent Peale (1952) and some psychologists prescribe the technique of visualization to those who want to bring about desired changes in their behaviour. For example, if a student finds it difficult to concentrate on a certain subject, he may be assigned the task of visualizing, that is, imagining a scene in which he is raptly concentrating on that very subject which is difficult for him to concentrate on. This kind of mental practice helps people to overcome their problems.

However, in REBT, the popular technique of imaging is used in a very innovative manner. Initially it was developed by Dr Maxie C. Maultsby, Jr. Dr Maultsby (1971) published a paper titled, 'Rational Emotive Imagery' in the journal, *Rational Living*. Almost immediately, Ellis realized that

Dr Maultsby's imagery technique was a very useful emotive one because it taught the client to get in touch with his disturbing emotions, then to intensify those emotions and finally change those emotions to healthy negative emotions. Hence, Ellis joined hands with Dr Maultsby and both of them developed the technique further. Maultsby and Ellis (1974) presented their refined version of imaging in the article 'Techniques for using Rational Emotive Imagery'. Subsequently, rational emotive imagery (REI) became one of the best emotive techniques in REBT.

REI consists of two parts. In the first part, the client is asked to imagine one of the incident when he was emotionally upset and what he felt at that time. (unhealthy emotion). He is encouraged to get in touch with his true emotion at that time and to experience it fully. In the second part, he is asked to imagine the same incident but has to replace the healthy emotion instead of unhealthy. REBT believes that in order to replace healthy emotions with unhealthy ones, the client has to change his underlying irrational self-talk. Hence, disputation occurs automatically. If the client practices REI once a day for a month, he gets habituated to replace healthy emotions in the place of unhealthy ones.

Let us see how Vikram can be helped by Ellis to resolve his problem by using this technique.

Ellis: Vikram, please sit comfortably and close your eyes. Now imagine that your boss has said something unpleasant to you and you are feeling angry at him. Yes, feel more and more angry at your boss.

Vikram: (After about 15 seconds) Yes, I am angry at my boss. In fact, I am very angry at my boss.

Ellis: Okay. Now concentrate on your anger and try to change it to a less disturbing and a more adaptable emotion. Try to feel somewhat annoyed but not angry.

Vikram: It is difficult.

Ellis: Yes, it is difficult. But try it. Make a genuine effort. Try to feel sorry and annoyed but not angry. There is no hurry. Try it patiently.

Vikram: (After about 25 seconds). Yes, I have changed my emotion of anger to annoyance.

Ellis: Good! How do you feel now?

Vikram: I am still uncomfortable. But this is better than feeling angry.

Ellis: All right! How did you change your anger to annoyance?

Vikram: I told myself something like, 'what my boss has said just now, doesn't have to trouble me excessively. My anger will not change my boss. Of course, I don't have to like him or what he has said. I can cope with him and what he has said'.

Ellis: Very good! Can you tell me why telling yourself those ideas helped you feel less upset?

Vikram: Perhaps those ideas prevented me from taking my boss and his remark too seriously. They gave a full stop to the insisting in my mind on how my boss *should* talk and behave.

Ellis: All right! Now go on doing this exercise everyday for about a month.

This excerpt of a therapy session, designed to teach REI to Vikram, is enough to show how the imaging technique is adapted and used in REBT.

However, it is necessary to emphasize that while using this technique, the therapist has two objectives in his mind. First, to help the client detect the more healthy emotion he would like to experience in a difficult situation. Second, to encourage the client to detect self-sentences and coping methods which are acceptable to him and then to practise them with REI so that they become his second nature.

Psychodrama

Psychodrama is one of those techniques which were used by psychotherapists long before REBT came into existence. Ellis does not hesitate to use techniques designed by different schools of psychotherapy, provided they can be fitted into the theoretical framework of REBT. This technique was originally developed by J. Moreno. It is a form of role playing in which the client is asked to play the role of another person with whom he faces the problem. It is an emotive-evocative technique and encourages the client to see his problem from the other person's perspectives.

Let us see how Ellis can use this technique with Vikram to achieve this basic objective of REBT. He enlists Vikram's co-operation for enacting a short play. In that play, Vikram plays the role of his boss, whereas Ellis plays the role of Vikram. The play is based on some episode described by Vikram, which reveals one of his unpleasant encounters with his boss.

Ellis (taking the role of Vikram) and Vikram playing the role of his boss, talk to each other for few minutes. Then Ellis asks Vikram to narrate his experience. The obvious purpose is to help Vikram detect the irrational beliefs about his boss. Ellis then encourages him to dispute those irrational beliefs. The procedure is repeated several times until Vikram feels comfortable with his newly learnt rational beliefs.

Reverse Role Play

This is a variation of Psychodrama. The purpose of this technique is to help a client who finds it difficult to dispute his own irrational beliefs.

In order to use this technique, Ellis will ask Vikram to play the role of Ellis, whereas Ellis will play the role of Vikram. They talk to each other according to their reversed roles. When Vikram plays Ellis' role, he is forced to detect and dispute his own irrational beliefs but temporarily adopted by his 'client' (his own). He is then forced to replace those irrational beliefs of his 'client' (his own) by alternative rational beliefs.

The technique of reverse role playing offers an excellent opportunity to the client to get fully involved in the work of uprooting irrational beliefs from his own mind and also replacing them with alternative rational beliefs.

Use of Humorous Techniques

In emotional disturbance, people generally lose the sense of humour. They tend to take things seriously. Due to this seriousness, people tend to magnify their problems. Ellis used a great deal of humour in the sessions to reduce this magnification and to dispel overly serious irrational thinking. Some of his favourite techniques were use of irony, absurdity, paradoxes, self-mocking or disputation of extreme awfulization, etc. Interestingly, he had presented a paper on how he used humour in REBT in symposium on humour at the APA Convention in Washington in 1976 (Ellis, 2001). He had mentioned many advantages of using humour for the clients. Some of them are as follows:

1. Humour helps you laugh at the behaviour of yourself and others, instead of seeing only the dark side.
2. It punctures your and others people's grandiosity.
3. It dramatically interrupts some of your dysfunctional patterns.
4. It shows you that human foibles are universal.

On realizing the importance of humour, it may be recalled that Ellis had himself composed many rational humorous songs intended to convey a rational philosophy of life to clients. It may be recalled that one of Ellis' popular humorous songs is presented in Box 8.1.

Let us see how Ellis will use humour in Vikram's case.

Vikram: 'My boss *must* not treat me unkindly and inconsiderably'.

Ellis: 'Yes, your boss *must* not do that because you run the universe and decide the rules of how boss *should* behave with their subordinates! How dare your boss to violate these rules? What a heinous crime to commit! He *should* have informed you that he is going to treat you unfairly and if you would have given him permission to do that, then and then only could he have ended his act! It is *horrible* to be treated unfairly because no one else in the world *ever* gets treated that way!'

It is seen from this dialogue that Ellis disputed Vikram's *must* and *awfulization* by using humorous techniques of irony, paradox and disputation of extreme awfulization.

Shame-attacking Exercises

Shortly after creating REBT and using it to treat his clients, Ellis observed that much of his clients' emotional disturbance consisted of their feelings of shame and embarrassment. They created these feelings in their minds when they felt that some of their behaviour was disgraceful according to them and others as well. However, that realization was not enough to make them feel ashamed. They felt ashamed when not only they put down their disgraceful behaviour but their entire personality for behaving in a disgraceful manner. Their feelings of shame and embarrassment were caused by their self-denigration. Moreover, their self-denigration was intense when they believed that other people had seen their unbecoming behaviour.

According to Ellis, human beings experience unhealthy emotions of shame and embarrassment when they berate themselves or their totality for their unseemly behaviour. On the contrary, if they only berate their poor behaviour or performance without devaluing themselves or their totality, they will create in their minds, healthy emotions of disappointment or sorrow about their behaviour.

To help his clients get rid of their feelings of shame and embarrassment, Ellis created shame-attacking exercises in 1968. These exercises consisted of giving some homework assignments to his clients which were likely to generate feelings of shame in their minds. For instance, they were asked to sing loudly in the street, to wear funny clothes, to read aloud the names of some shops in the street, etc. Such exercises were designed to teach them that although their behaviour could be laughable or even stupid, they themselves could not be called justifiably stupid persons. In short, the shame-attacking exercises are intended to teach clients to accept themselves unconditionally in spite of their laughable, unseemly or stupid behaviour.

Let us look at Vikram's problem. Of course, he is angry at his boss. He may be creating feelings of shame in his mind for being insulted in front of his colleagues. In that case, Ellis would first help him get rid of his feelings of shame before helping him get rid of his anger at his boss. To achieve this objective, he may ask Vikram to tell his close friends and relatives how querulously he becomes oversensitive to the insult and thereby invites the ridicule and criticism of many of his colleagues in his department. If Vikram is ridiculed and criticized by his friends and relatives for his querulous behaviour, Ellis encourages him to accept the fact that he is feeling intense shame for being ridiculed. Then, he teaches him to accept himself unconditionally in spite of his unbecoming behaviour vis-à-vis his boss and in spite of being ridiculed and criticized by his friends and relatives for frequently getting hurt by his boss' comments.

Self-disclosure

This technique was used by Ellis to show his clients that sometimes he also made himself emotionally disturbed and that he was not ashamed of telling them about his own emotional disturbance. In fact, he made it known to them that because of his rational philosophy of life, he accepted himself in spite of his emotional upsets. Thus, he modelled a rational philosophy of life by openly disclosing his own shortcomings.

Suppose the REBT therapist is dealing with a client who is feeling extremely anxious about going to hospital for a medical check-up. The therapist does not hesitate to disclose how at one time, he too felt very anxious about going to hospital for a medical check-up and how he accepted himself with his anxiety and then used REBT to cope with his anxiety. This technique strengthens the rapport between the therapist and the client. It also motivates the client to apply REBT to solve his emotional problem by using REBT.

Can Ellis use this technique to treat Vikram? Yes, he would narrate the situation when he was working in 'Distinctive Creations', a gift shop, as assistant accountant. That was the era of Great Depression. He got the job with a lot of effort. He thought that his boss was exploiting him. However, he could not leave the job due to the scarcity of jobs available in the market.

Ellis would disclose to Vikram how he used to get angry towards his boss and when he realized that his resentment was not helping him to achieve the goal, how he brought a change in his beliefs and how he moved towards the healthy feeling of annoyance instead of anger with the help of REBT. He would also describe eventually how he was successful in winning the confidence of his boss and getting a promotion later on. As a result, he served this company for 10 years and completed his PhD in the tenure.

Other Techniques

Some other emotive techniques were also used by Ellis. For instance, he judiciously made use of some selected mottoes, parables, humorous episodes and songs, aphorisms, inspirational quotes, etc. In the case of Vikram, Ellis may suggest some mottoes or slogans to him with a view to helping him get rid of his anger. Followings are three such mottoes:

1. Anger creates more harm to you than your enemy.
2. Nobody can insult you without your permission.
3. You become what you hate.

Some other useful emotive slogans are mentioned in Box 9.2.

Box 9.2

Examples of Useful Emotive Slogans

1. Do not fix the blame; fix the problem.
2. To err proves human; to forgive leaves you sane and realistic.
3. You can make good things happen out of most bad things.
4. No gain without pain.
5. Strike while the iron is hot.
6. This too will pass.
7. When you are listless, you may become listless.
8. Today: Use it or lose it.
9. Well begun is half done.
10. Press on!
11. If you do not stand for something, you will fall for anything.
12. To be needy is to be bleedy.

(Box 9.2 Continued)

(Box 9.2 Continued)

13. Doing gets it done.
14. Adversity is a blessing in disguise.
15. Do the doable.
16. Doing beats stewing.
17. People who take too much care go nowhere.
18. Accept and cope rather than condemn and mope.
19. Have a happy tomorrow; do today's work today.
20. Do it or ditch it.

Behavioural Techniques

Although REBT mainly focuses on changing the client's irrational philosophy of life, it does not rely only on cognitive techniques to achieve this objective. We have seen how REBT uses a number of emotive techniques to supplement its cognitive techniques for achieving its main objective. However, it does not stop there. As thinking, feeling and behaving are intrinsically integrated and holistic processes, REBT also uses many behavioural techniques to supplement these two types of techniques. Moreover, it is known that behavioural changes expedite cognitive changes.

Incidentally, it is important to bear in mind that Ellis was practising as a marital and sex therapist before he invented REBT. Even at that time, he used to give behavioural assignments to his clients, which they were supposed to carry out between therapy sessions.

Therefore, let us try to understand some important behavioural techniques used in REBT. To make this work somewhat easy, we shall turn our attention to Saniya, our third case, and see how Ellis can help her by using some behavioural techniques. Of course, we shall presume that Ellis has already demolished the depression-creating irrational belief in her mind by using some cognitive and emotive techniques before supplementing his work by adopting some behavioural techniques.

Reinforcements and Penalties

As many eminent behaviourists, like B.F. Skinner, have shown that behaviour which is rewarded (reinforced) is strengthened, whereas behaviour which is punished (penalized) is extinguished. In REBT, this basic principle is used to shape the behaviour of clients.

Analysis of Case 5.3 in Light of Behavioural Techniques

Can Ellis use this technique to treat Saniya? Yes, he can ask her which activity she finds enjoyable. Suppose she enjoys watching television, then Ellis gives her an assignment. Her assignment is to enjoy watching television if she has followed the diet prescribed by her doctor with the intention of reducing her weight by 5 kg. Hence, watching television becomes reinforcement for the behaviour of implementing the prescribed diet. This kind of reinforcement makes her task of dieting somewhat pleasant. Ellis also tells her that if she fails to follow the prescribed diet, she has to forego the pleasure of watching television. In this way, pleasurable activities are used to strengthen desirable behaviour.

Though reinforcement and penalties are behavioural activities, they have cognitive and emotive components too. Saniya gets pleasure from watching television. She tells herself that it is worth to follow the prescribed diet for this pleasure. She is motivated by her thoughts (cognition) and desire (emotion).

Further, Ellis collaborates with Saniya in order to decide which activity can be used as a penalty for her not behaving in a desirable manner, that is, not following the prescribed diet. Suppose she dislikes washing her clothes. Ellis then gives her another assignment. Her assignment is to wash her clothes if she fails to follow the prescribed diet. The purpose of this assignment is to induce her to follow even the difficult schedule of a diet so as to avoid the unpleasant task of washing clothes.

Ellis can combine the technique of reinforcement and the technique of penalty. For instance, he can ask Saniya to forego the enjoyment of watching television and to wash her clothes when she does not follow the prescribed diet.

However, it requires being emphasized that in REBT, reinforcements and penalties are used to encourage the client to inculcate a rational cost-benefit philosophy. For example, Ellis will expect Saniya to learn the philosophy that in the long run it is costly not to follow the prescribed diet because it will entail foregoing some pleasure in life and/or incurring some unpleasant consequences. Although it is hard to follow the prescribed diet in the short run, it is beneficial in the long run. This understanding will help her acquire and maintain the philosophy of HFT.

Risk Taking

Many clients refrain from socializing because they are afraid of being rejected by others. Of course, this is not the only reason why people don't undertake activities that they consider risky. Often the activities they fear are not very risky. For example, some clients avoid using elevators or escalators. Some others avoid learning how to swim even under the guidance of a professional trainer. Some do not dare to go to college for getting a university degree. In reality, the risks involved in such activities are not terrible or awful. Since, clients who are afraid of those activities never undertake them, they deprive themselves of the opportunities to get rid of their anxiety.

While dealing with such anxious clients, the REBT therapist gives them the assignment of doing those dreaded activities. His purpose is to help them realize that the activities they are afraid of are not so dangerous, and some of those activities are even enjoyable.

Suppose Saniya is afraid to implement the prescribed diet because she believes that if she begins to follow it and after some days goofs and begins to eat and drink indiscriminately, her relatives and friends will laugh at her. In order to deal with this anxiety, Ellis will ask her to start implementing the prescribed diet and after getting used to it, one day deliberately take the risk of eating and drinking indiscriminately in the presence of her relatives and friends and expose herself to the possibility of being ridiculed by them.

Ellis' next step will be to show Saniya that the disapproval of others is not terrible or awful as she thought; it is just annoying and disappointing. Similarly, even if she fails to maintain her perfect record of following the prescribed diet once in a while, she does not become a worthless person. Therefore, she can accept herself with her imperfect record as well as the disapproval of others.

This technique is quite similar to the technique of giving shame-attacking exercises to the clients. The only difference is that in shame-attacking exercises, the probability of being rejected by others is more. Besides, they are obviously meant for clients who are prone to make themselves feel ashamed and embarrassed. The point to note is that risk-taking exercises are intended to help clients overcome their irrational philosophy of awfulization and self-downing.

Acting on Rational Beliefs

In REBT, clients are taught not to behave according to their irrational beliefs; instead, they are urged to replace those beliefs by alternative rational beliefs and behave accordingly. One effective way of bringing about such changes in clients is to ask them to push themselves consciously to behave as though they hold only rational beliefs. This technique is particularly useful when clients agree to behave rationally only when they will feel inspired to do so. On the contrary, the therapist persuades them to behave rationally whether they feel inspired to behave sensibly or not.

If Saniya is planning to follow the prescribed diet when she feels inspired to do so on her birthday, Ellis urges her to begin the programme of eating and drinking according to the prescribed diet immediately. Here, the idea is that efforts to implement the prescribed diet will bring about a change in her irrational thinking and inspire her to continue to do the undertaken task.

Staying in Difficult Situations

When clients feel anxious in some vulnerable situations, they tend to avoid those situations. Hence, the REBT therapist gives them exercise of staying in a very difficult situation and practising not making themselves upset about it. The rationale behind this exercise is that when the clients get enough practice of not making themselves upset about difficult situation, they no more feel it difficult rather they welcome it.

Suppose, even after getting used to following the prescribed diet, Saniya avoids going to parties because she may be tempted to eat and drink indiscriminately. Ellis will then ask her to go to parties and enjoy the company of those who eat and drink merrily. This will help her inculcate and strengthen the philosophy of HFT. Besides, even if she eats and drinks by disregarding the prescribed diet once in a while, Ellis will teach her to accept herself unconditionally and without awfulizing about her lapse.

Paradoxical Homework

This technique was originally developed by Viktor Frankl (1959) and since then many therapists are using it in their sessions. By using this technique, an REBT therapist assigns the task of doing what they really want to stop doing. Clients who want to give up the habit of worrying are asked by the therapist to go on worrying almost continually for a week or so. Similarly, clients who are perfectionists and therefore afraid of committing mistakes are asked by the therapist to deliberately make mistakes in their daily activities. If clients want to overcome their depression, the therapist will ask them to make themselves more and more depressed. This will help them to view their problems from a different perspective and do some reality testing.

Ellis may ask Saniya to attend parties and deliberately eat and drink to her heart's content in the company of her relatives and friends and then feel more depressed. She will find it difficult to carry out this assignment and make herself more depressed. In fact, she will realize that she used to trouble herself by telling herself, 'I *must* not eat and drink indiscriminately, and I *must* not feel depressed'.

Of course, if Saniya does eat and drink to her heart's content and feel depressed, Ellis will teach her to accept herself unconditionally without blaming herself for her own self-harming behaviour and unhealthy emotion of depression.

Skill Training

Some clients may learn to replace their irrational beliefs by alternative rational beliefs. However, they don't have the skills necessary for scheduling and carrying out their daily activities including dieting. Such clients are taught some skills required for effectively implementing their newly acquired philosophy of life.

Suppose Saniya is afraid that her relatives and friends may laugh at her and make some adverse comments about her failure to follow the prescribed diet consistently. This idea will make her feel anxious and depressed. In order to help her cope with such a situation, Ellis will not only show her that she does not become a worthless person because of her failure to follow the prescribed diet consistently but also teach her to accept herself unconditionally with her failure. Further, he will teach her some social skills so that she can cope with the adverse comments of others assertively without blaming them or herself.

A few examples of behavioural assignment are stated in Table 9.1.

Table 9.1

A Few Examples of Behavioural Assignment

No.	Behavioural Assignment
1.	*Reading Assignment*
	Reading some valuable literature on REBT: theory and practice will help you to gain insights on REBT practice. For example, you can read Chapters 4, 5 and 6 of this book to become familiar with the ABC model.
2.	*Writing Assignment*
	The 3-2-1 reflection exercise is a good example of writing assignment. When you read the above chapters or learn some principle of REBT, write down the following points on a piece of paper:
	• 3 things I learned today
	• 2 things I need to focus on
	• 1 thing I practise immediately
	This exercise will help you to gain conceptual clarity on REBT and to implement your learnings into practice. Self-help homework sheets, written essays and log books are other examples of written assignments.
3.	*Action Assignment*
	Action assignment will push you to work in a difficult situation and revaluate your definition of certain behaviours as terribly dangerous. For example, collect three rejections in one week or to do something what others do not appreciate.

Effective Philosophy of Life

Analysis of Cases 5.1, 5.2 and 5.3 in Reference to the Effective Philosophy of Life

If Aditi, Vikram and Saniya seek Ellis' help to reduce their emotional disturbance, they would acquire the effective philosophy of life. At this stage, Ellis would work on their philosophic restructuring to change their dysfunctional personalities. On following steps (Ellis, 1976, p. 29), he would check the progress:

1. They can fully acknowledge that we create, to a lesser or greater extent, our own disturbances.
2. They can see clearly that we do have the ability to change these disturbances significantly.

3. They understand that what we usually call 'emotional problems' stem mainly from irrational beliefs.
4. They clearly perceive these beliefs and dispute them.
5. They realize that they would better work hard in emotive and behavioural ways to counteract these beliefs and the unhealthy feelings and actions to which they lead.
6. They reuse and re-practice rational-emotive behavioural methods of uprooting and changing disturbed consequences for the rest of their lives.

This restricting will not only help them to solve their current emotional problems but will also motivate them to change their underlying faulty cognitions, ideas, beliefs or philosophies of life. They will be able to see their self-defeating views, learn to question, challenge them and change them for more self-helping outlooks. They will get rid of unhealthy emotions and try to inculcate healthy emotions instead. They will act according to their newly acquired healthy outlook. In short, the attainment of effective philosophy of life will bring an elegant transformation in their thoughts, emotions and behaviour.

Some Important Caveats

We have taken a brief overview of some important therapeutic techniques used in REBT. Of course, practitioners of REBT use many other techniques while treating their clients. However, it is necessary to bring home to the readers the following crucial points about the practice of REBT:

1. Although the techniques used in REBT are classified under three heads, namely, cognitive, emotive and behavioural, no technique is purely cognitive, emotive or behavioural. As cognitive, emotive and behavioural processes are not disparate, rather they are interrelated, interactive and holistic processes. Therefore, our classification of techniques is somewhat arbitrary. Let us take the example of shame-attacking exercises. In this book, the technique is listed under the category 'Emotive Techniques'. However, it can be listed under the category, 'Behavioural Techniques' too.
2. We have presumed that each of our three cases cling to only one musturbatory ideology, and is disturbed by only one unhealthy emotion. However, in reality, most of the clients are disturbed

by many unhealthy emotions as they cling to more than one musturbatory ideologies.

That is the reason why Aditi may feel angry at the interviewers and depressed as well if she fails to get the job she wants. Similarly, Vikram can feel ashamed because of being insulted by his boss in front of others. Saniya can feel anxious about the comments of her relatives and friends.

3. It would be a gross misconception to believe that Aditi can be helped by only using cognitive techniques; Vikram can be treated by using only emotive techniques; and Saniya can be induced to follow the prescribed diet by using only behavioural techniques. As a matter of fact, REBT practitioners use a combination of cognitive, emotive and behavioural techniques with almost any client.

4. If the client is having the secondary emotional disturbance about his primary emotional disturbance, the therapist first helps him get rid of his secondary emotional disturbance, and then he turns his attention to the primary emotional disturbance.

For example, Aditi is anxious about the job interview. Ellis notices that she is also creating in her mind the secondary emotional disturbance of depression, guilt and self-pity. Hence, he will first help her to reduce her secondary emotional disturbance and then to get rid of her primary emotional disturbance, that is, anxiety.

Similarly, if the client, after becoming aware of his secondary emotional disturbance, creates a tertiary emotional disturbance about his secondary emotional disturbance, the therapist will first help him to reduce his tertiary emotional disturbance. Then the therapist will then help him to reduce his secondary emotional disturbance. Finally, he will help the client tackle his primary emotional disturbance.

5. While describing the techniques used in REBT, it is presumed that the therapist is dealing with an individual client. Like most other systems of psychotherapy, REBT is useful for helping groups of clients as well. A group may consist of two people (like husband and wife) or more people, but usually not more than about 12–14 people. In other words, just as the therapist can do individual therapy, he can also do group therapy for helping a small group of clients. While offering group therapy, the therapist uses more or less the same techniques that he uses for doing individual therapy. However, the exact methodology of doing group therapy is beyond the scope of this book.

Hopefully, these five crucial points will give you a deeper insight into the nature of an REBT practitioner's day-to-day work.

References

Dryden, W. (1986). A case of theoretically consistent eclecticism: Humanizing a computer addict. *International Journal of Eclectic Psychotherapy, 5*(4), 309–27.

Ellis, A. (1976). Toward a new theory of personality. In A. Ellis, & J.M. Whiteley (Eds.), *Theoretical and Empirical Foundations of Rational-Emotive Therapy* (p. 29). Monterey, CA: Brooks/Cole.

———. (1977). *Anger: How to Live With and Without* (p. 56). New York: Readers Digest Press.

———. (2000). *How to Control Your Anxiety Before It Controls You.* New York: Citadel Press/Kensington Publishing Corp.

———. (2001). *Feeling Better, Getting Better, Staying Better: Profound Self-Help Therapy for Your Emotions* (p. 159). Atascadero, CA: Impact Publishers.

Ellis, A., & Harper, R.A. (1997). *A Guide to Rational Living* (3rd Rev. ed.). North Hollywood, CA: Melvin Powers.

Frankl, V. (1959). *Man's Search for Meaning* (1984 ed., p. 126). New York: NY: Simon & Schuster.

Maultsby, M.C., Jr (1971). Rational Emotive Imagery. *Rational Living, 6*(1), 24–27.

Maultsby, M.C., Jr & Ellis, A. (1974). *Techniques for Using Rational-Emotive Imagery.* New York, NY: Institute for Rational-Emotive Therapy.

Peale, N.V. (1952). *The Power of Positive Thinking.* New York: Prentice-Hall Inc.

Phadke, K.M. (1968–2003). *Albert Ellis Papers* [Series I: Correspondence, 1947–2006], Correspondence of K.M. Phadke & Dr. Albert Ellis, Columbia University Libraries Archival Collection. http://findingaids.cul.columbia.edu/ead/nnc-rb/ldpd_8683406/dsc/1

Further Readings

Dryden, W. (1990). *Rational-Emotive Counselling in Action.* New Delhi: SAGE.

Ellis, A. (1993). Rational-emotive imagery: RET version. In M.E. Bernard & J.L. Wolfe (Eds.), *The RET Resource Book for Practitioners* (pp. II8–II10). New York: Institute for Rational-Emotive Therapy.

———. (2004). *Rational Emotive Behavior Therapy: It Works For Me – It Can Work For You.* New York, NY: Prometheus books.

Phadke, K.M. (1999). *Adhunik Sanjivani.* Mumbai: Tridal Prakashan.

10

Applications of REBT

Today, REBT is widely recognized as an effective approach to psychotherapy. In the last 60 years, it has widened its scope so much that it is applied extensively to almost every walk of life. It has contributed significantly to various fields such as social science, education, industry, healthcare, sexology, family and marital field, dieting, sports and others. These contributions are so valuable that not only psychologists but also researchers from other areas acknowledge it.

REBT is also used for a broad range of mental health problems. Emotional disturbance makes people feel unhappy and tends to adversely affect their performance in almost any field of activity. Therefore, REBT can be effectively used to help them reduce their unhappiness and improve their overall performance. Ellis himself has written a number of articles and books to show how REBT can be useful to those who have emotional problems related to fatal illness, physical disabilities, dying and death, fear of flying, inferiority complex, procrastination, and so on, you name it. Here, we shall consider REBT applications to some of the major fields. Hopefully, a careful study of those applications of REBT will help you understand how it may be used in other spheres of life.

Sexology

One of the most important subjects in which Ellis' rebelliousness against the conventional ideas and practices is prominently visible is sexology. Therefore, it is befitting to begin our broad survey of applications of REBT to some selected sexual problems. Of course, we shall not only cover the subject of sexology but also related subjects such as love, marriage and family therapy. Another reason for beginning with this subject is that

Ellis began practising as a marriage, family and sex therapist long before he invented REBT.

In an article, Ellis (1977) frankly states that he began to take interest in sex when he was a five-year-old boy. His serious interest in the subject of love and sex can be traced back to the period in his life when he was 26 years old. During that period, he decided to write some non-fiction (i.e., something serious or scholarly) about love and sex. This was not an abrupt or understandable decision, of course. Since the age of 12, he had entertained the ambition of becoming a writer. When he was 18, he began to write novels, poems and plays and by the time he was 28, he had completed 20 or so book-length manuscripts—novels, poems, etc.—many of which were quite provocative. Unfortunately, no publisher was willing to accept any of his literary output. As a result, he arrived at the decision that he would write something serious and useful about love, sex, marriage, etc. that might be published and sold. This decision was strengthened by his genuine interest in these subjects.

For two years, he read hundreds of books, articles, etc. on sex, love and marriage. As a result, his friends and relatives gradually came to know that he had become some sort of an expert on sex and related subjects. They began to discuss their problems regarding sex and love with him and Ellis could give them some useful advice. Encouraged by the feedback he received from his friends and relatives, Ellis decided to become a counsellor. In fact, he established the LAMP Institute. However, his enthusiasm was somewhat dampened when his lawyer warned him about legal troubles of practising as a psychotherapist without the necessary qualifications and accreditation. His determination was so strong that he obtained a PhD degree in clinical psychology from Columbia University and became a professional clinical psychologist in 1947. All this account is a brief summary of what is narrated at length in Chapter 2 of this book, 'Life and Development'.

Once Ellis became a professional psychotherapist, he made further valuable contributions to his favourite field, that is, sex, love and marriage. He enriched the science of sexology and related subjects by doing research, offering therapy to clients and educating the people by giving lectures, workshops and writing articles and books. Suffice it to say that, in due course, these multifaceted efforts earned for him the reputation of being one of the foremost authorities on love and sex in the world. Besides, many professional societies bestowed upon him their prestigious awards. In fact, his achievements in his favourite field are too numerous to summarize briefly. Therefore, it is enough to mention that he is one of the founders of the Society for Scientific Study of Sex and was its first president.

Ironically enough, these achievements are of a scholar who was practically forced to give up the plan of doing his PhD thesis on the love emotions of college women by the ultraconservative powers at Columbia University. Of course, on the basis of whatever research he had done before switching to a non-controversial subject for his PhD thesis, Ellis published several articles in some reputed professional journals.

The contributions Ellis made to the field of sex, love and marriage and family after obtaining his PhD in clinical psychology are so multifarious that any attempt to present even a sketchy account of it is a formidable task. These contributions are founded on his extensive and intensive study of existing knowledge, personal experience of love and sex, scientific research and vast clinical experience.

Scientific Research on Sex

It is worth recalling that even before doing any scientific research and acquiring clinical experience, Ellis had done a good deal of library research into sexology and related subjects. On the basis of his painstaking research, he had written a book titled *The Case for Sexual Promiscuity.* This title of the book itself announced that the contents of his book were definitely rebellious. In the 1940s, even American publishers had found the book too risky to publish. Subsequently, only the first part of the book was published in 1965 under the title, *The Case for Sexual Liberty* (Ellis, 1965a).

However, Ellis' most significant scientific research on love, sex and marriage culminated in the book, *The Folklore of Sex* (Ellis, 1951). Again, it was not easy for Ellis to get a publisher for this book. He had to overcome several obstacles before the book was published in 1951 by Doubleday and Company. Some people were unhappy with the publishing house and about the book's liberal attitudes towards sex. It began to be known to laymen only after its revised paperback edition was published by Grover Press in 1962.

Ellis' major objective of the research project on which the book was based was clear-cut. He wanted to investigate which beliefs about sex and related subjects were commonly held by the American people in the mid-1950s. In order to understand the beliefs about sex and love prevalent during this period, Ellis gathered relevant information from a cross-section of newspapers, journals, magazines, films, popular songs, radio and television shows, etc., available on 1 January 1950.

After carefully studying the collected information, Ellis found that sexual practices prevailing among the American people were different from the lofty ideals preached by religious, political and educational leaders. For instance, some organizations were committed to the cause of wiping out venereal diseases. Yet, in practice, they were against demanding mass examination and treatment of venereal diseases. These organizations were not consistent in their avowed beliefs and actual practices.

The data collected by Ellis clearly showed that sex in advertisements, jokes, etc. were very popular among the masses. However, it was frowned upon by censoring authorities. As a good researcher, Ellis not only presented the facts revealed by his empirical investigation but also made interpretative comments on those facts. According to him, if the guardians of American morality did not grumble and reproach the sexual desires and acts openly expressed in the media, perhaps the sexuality deviantly expressed in stories, pin-up photographs, etc. might not have become as popular as it obviously was in the mid-1950s. He also believed that prudish attitudes and senseless censorship in relation to sexual intercourse proved to be harmful because they gave rise to a pathological behaviour that forced the normal desires to follow the law-breaking and guilt-producing secrecy.

It is significant to note that while commenting on these views of Ellis, his first biographer, Dr Daniel N. Wiener (1988), remarks that ironically enough, in the mid-1980s, the American public believed that the sexual troubles in their society were created by too much permissiveness! Although, the sexual troubles in their society were not different when censorship and rigidity were listed as its prime causes.

When Dr Daniel N. Wiener asked Ellis to comment on this irony in an interview in 1985, Ellis did not budge. On the contrary, he said that even 35 years after his interpretative comments on the facts he collected, the American society had remained as conservative as before, in the sense that it still harped on the same theme: love and sex *must* go together; nudity *must* be banned; reduce inhibition only in pornography (which, anyway, is often misleading in other ways).

Yet, another conclusion Ellis drew from his study was that in the American society, conservative attitude towards sex was ruling except in plays, humour and men's magazines. He further added that practically all Americans were muddled and messed up as far as their views about sex were concerned. Of course, they often kept on changing their views. They enjoyed those sex acts the most which they thought were not proper. At the same time, if they did not indulge in those sex acts, they felt tensed and uncomfortable! Hence, by and large, the result was hypocrisy, evasion and out-and-out lying.

Under the circumstances, what alternatives were available to the American people? They could either follow the consistently liberal path in their ideas about and practices of sex behaviour or follow strictly the path of conservative ideas about and practices of sex behaviour. However, both the paths are dangerous because they will invite the American people to adopt a lifestyle different from their current lifestyle. Indeed, this is a difficult choice!

The second part of Ellis' earlier research-based book, *The Folklore of Sex* (Ellis, 1951), was published in 1954 as *The American Sexual Tragedy* (Ellis, 1954). In the second part, Ellis sums up the American people's attitudes towards specific topics such as love, marriage and family relations. His observation is that to a certain extent, sexual satisfaction of men and women is impaired due to the existing social attitudes towards non-coital sex relations. Moreover, the puritanical views about sex were responsible for the unimaginable misery prevailing in love, marriage and family relations.

Ellis' findings also revealed that sex and love relations among the American people were not damaged by the problems created by individuals; rather, they were caused by socially created taboos and norms. Therefore, according to him, unless some drastic changes in the social attitudes and norms were effected, sex and love relations would not become more open and fulfilling. Incidentally, he does not fail to recall that the Kinsey et al. (1948, 1953) findings had also pointed out the necessity of revising sex attitudes in order to achieve sexual sanity.

These views were expressed by Ellis in the mid-1950s. Have not the American people's attitudes towards sex and related subjects become far more liberal in the past 60 years or so? If so, have those liberal attitudes brought more sexual sanity in America? All that one can honestly say regarding these two questions is that these are not at all easy to answer!

Is there any other significant example of Ellis' research work in the area of human sexuality? Yes, one may point out to an article he contributed to the book, *Sex, Society, and the Individual* (Pillay & Ellis, 1953). This book was edited by Dr Pillay and Ellis himself. Dr Pillay was the editor of *The International Journal of Sexology*, which, at that time, was published in Mumbai, India. The book contains 45 articles contributed by scholars. Three of those articles were contributed by Ellis himself.

One among the three articles contributed by Ellis was titled, 'A Study of 300 Sex Offenders'. The very title of the article gives the impression that apparently it was based on some empirical research. Indeed, it was. What did Ellis say about sex offenders? According to him, sex offenders, except rapists, usually did not use force. Of course, they often showed psychological disturbance. They were not too dangerous or impulsive criminals. However, Ellis presented no specific theoretical hypothesis regarding the causes of sex offences. Nor did he offer any guidelines for offering therapy to sex offenders.

Enduring Contributions

Self-help books: Ellis wanted to liberate the people from irrational ideas about sex. Hence, he enlightened people on many sexual topics by his forthright writing. He went on examining the social attitudes towards oral and anal intercourse, and the guilt associated with sex, etc. As a result, Ellis wrote many books on sex and related topics meant for the laymen. Those books may be described as self-help or how-to-do manuals. The titles of some of those books are quite self-explanatory: *The Art and Science of Love* (Ellis, 1960), *The Sensuous Person* (Ellis, 1972c), *Sex and the Liberated Man* (Ellis, 1976).

Three of his very popular books deserve a special mention. First, *Sex and the Single Man* (Ellis, 1963b). The book begins by describing the price one has to pay for sexual abstinence. The message is clear. Even if you decide not to marry and remain single all your life, you had better not deprive yourself of sexual gratification. The book then gives you techniques for finding out a suitable partner and enjoy life.

If you are avoiding marriage because of fears, the book teaches you how to overcome them. Finally, if you decide to marry, the book offers you many techniques of proposing to the person of your choice and then living your life happily though you are married!

The second book that deserves to be specifically mentioned is entitled *The Intelligent Woman's Guide to Man Hunting* (Ellis, 1963). It was revised and published under the new title, *The Intelligent Woman's Guide to Dating and Mating* (Ellis, 1979). Written in a humorous style, the book encourages women to be more assertive in the pursuit of a suitable partner. In fact, the third chapter in the book was entitled 'How to Become Assertive Without Being Aggressive'. The book can also be considered as one of the pioneering books on assertiveness training. In 1949, Andrew Salter (1949) had published the book, *Conditioned Reflex Therapy*, which also taught its readers how to be assertive in dealing with others.

The third book which requires a special mention is *The Civilized Couple's Guide to Extramarital Adventures* (Ellis, 1972b). This book is a response to the well-documented fact that extramarital liaisons exist and suggests how to tackle them. Of course, it is not correct to consider it as just another how-to-do book on love and sex. It is certainly more than that because it raises some basic moral questions. Therefore, we will have more to say about Ellis' views on sexual morality later.

Other contributions: Besides writing self-help books on love and sex for the interested laymen, Ellis has authored and edited many articles and books which contain some lasting contributions to sexology and related subjects. Therefore, we shall address ourselves to some of those important contributions.

Clitoral orgasm: Freud and many of his followers believed that women were capable of experiencing two quite different kinds of orgasms: clitoral orgasm and vaginal orgasm. It was also believed that clitoral orgasm was experienced by girls and young women and it represented an immature sexual reaction. When young women grew up and matured, they replaced the inferior and immature sexual reaction of clitoral orgasm by a more mature (and presumably superior) sexual reaction, that is, vaginal orgasm. Afterwards many psychologists, psychiatrists and sexologists challenged that Freudian view and went to the extent of propounding the theory that the vaginal orgasm was a myth. According to this new theory, if women achieved orgasm, no matter how, it was a legitimate and mature sexual reaction. The controversy continued for many years.

Ellis was one of the few professionals who never believed in the Freudian theory of two different types of orgasms. Hence, Ellis (1963a) published a paper and brilliantly reviewed both sides of the controversy and drew many important and balanced conclusions.

According to Ellis, women can enjoy vaginal and non-vaginal stimulation. Clitoral and vaginal satisfaction need not be mutually exclusive. Women can be gratified in both ways. Moreover, men and women had better keep their minds open to the fact that just as sexual satisfaction includes physical sensations, it is influenced by many attitudinal factors. So far, as orgasmic and non-orgasmic sexual reactions are concerned, women show very wide individual differences.

Ellis was one of the few psychoanalysts who were foremost in attacking the Freudian theory of the immaturity and inferiority of the clitoral orgasm.

Ellis' views in the mentioned paper are almost universally accepted by today's sexologists and sex therapists.

Encyclopaedia: Let us now turn to one of the major contributions Ellis made to the field of sexology. In collaboration with Dr Albert Abarbanel, Ellis edited a massive two volumes *Encyclopedia of Sexual Behaviour* (Ellis & Abarbanel, 1961). It contained authoritative articles on different topics contributed by more than one hundred experts, including Ellis. It was considered as a comprehensive and standard reference book on sexology and was very well received in many countries besides the United States of America.

Of course, Ellis was ideally qualified to edit and publish the encyclopaedia with a renowned scholar such as Albert Abarbanel. When Ellis undertook the gigantic work, he had already authored well over 20 books on sex, love and marriage. The revised edition of the encyclopaedia was published in 1974 and, for many following years, it was considered the most comprehensive and reliable reference book on sex and related topics. Of course, all such scholarly books became outdated over a long period of time. Naturally, the encyclopaedia is not as up-to-date today as it was several decades ago. Nevertheless, it cannot be denied that Ellis and Dr Albert Abarbanel made a monumental contribution to sexology by publishing the two-volume reference book.

Now we turn our attention to what Ellis has to say about other sex-related topics on the basis of his vast clinical and personal experience as well as his up-to-date knowledge of other sexologists' contributions to the topics we are discussing.

Masturbation

Masturbation is one of the few topics on which Ellis' rebelliousness reaches its peak. His rebellious views on a few other topics made him notorious in the late 1950s. It may be recalled that he discovered masturbation and then began to practise it when he was a 12-year-old boy. By the time he was 15 years old, he used to masturbate twice a day but without feeling guilty. He thought that he perhaps lacked self-control. Therefore, he read a lot of books on sex in the public library and found that some authors assured their readers that there was nothing wrong in masturbation even when it was done frequently. When Ellis grew up, he thought that those books were quite good in view of the fact that they were published in the 1920s.

No doubt, in the following decades, views about masturbation became more liberal and many distinguished writers consoled their readers that masturbation was not as bad as it was once thought to be. Ellis' message was far more radical and he wanted to present it in a frank and forthright style. Hence, in an article, Ellis (1956a) declared that 'it is difficult to conceive of a more beneficial, harmless, tension-releasing human act than masturbation that is spontaneously performed without (puritanically-inculcated and actually groundless) fears and anxiety'. However, it was not easy for Ellis to get the article published in a professional journal. Dr A.P. Pillay (whom we have met earlier), the editor of the *International Journal of Sexology*, which was published in Mumbai, India, refused to accept it, although Ellis was the American editor of the journal. Dr A.P. Pillay felt that Ellis' outspoken article might offend some people belonging to certain sectarian groups in India. Subsequently, the article was published by the iconoclastic periodical, *The Independent*, in the year 1956.

Here is another example of how Ellis's forthright views on masturbation were unacceptable even to a professional journal. The editor of *The Journal of Social Therapy* requested Ellis to write an article on masturbation among prisoners. The journal was the official publication of the Medical Correctional Association. Yet, when Ellis' article was published, he was shocked to see that the most important paragraph in his article was totally omitted! What was the gist of censored paragraph? It stated that prison authorities *should* not discourage the prisoners under their control from masturbating. Instead, they had better be thankful that some normal outlet for the sexual urge was available to the captives under their control. Ellis was so convinced about his conclusion that he later published a book entitled *The Psychology of Sex Offenders* (Ellis, 1956b), based on his actual work with prisoners' and research findings.

These examples are intended to show how Ellis being a rebellious psychologist had difficulties in getting his writings published. One can go on enumerating several obstacles he had to overcome in order to get his subsequent books on sex published. Hence, it is not necessary to do so. Suffice it to say that his efforts to be honest about the subject of sex met with strong opposition from publishers, editors, lawyers and many readers too. Therefore, he advised authors who want to write about sex. His advice only repeats the famous Punch magazine gave well over a century ago to men wanting to marry: Don't!

Back to Ellis' paper (1956a), 'New Light on Masturbation'. What did he say in that paper which was found so shocking and repulsive by the then orthodoxy? First, he considered all the objections against masturbation and refuted them one by one on the basis of scientific knowledge and clinical experience. The main objections he took into account were as follows: masturbation is immature and unsocial; it does not lead to full emotional satisfaction; it is sexually frustrating; it leads to impotence or frigidity; and finally, it leads to sexual excess.

If Ellis were to restrict the scope of his paper to refuting objections against masturbation and showing that it was not injurious to man's body and mind, he might not have met with as much opposition as he did. However, He went further and taught people that masturbation, far from being harmful, was an excellent tension-reducing and joy-producing act. This was unacceptable to his opponents.

However, Ellis was not going to placate his adversaries in his subsequent writings on masturbation. In his book, *Sex and the Liberated Man*, Ellis (1976) wrote a full chapter entitled 'The Art and Science of Masturbation'. In this chapter, he again refutes all major objections against masturbation and then goes on to describe 21 advantages of masturbation. Further, he even goes to the extent of teaching several specific techniques of masturbation.

In the following decades, social norms and values underwent great changes, and Ellis' rebellious views got acceptance from scholars in sexology and common man as well. When Manfred DeMartino edited the comprehensive book *Human Autoerotic Practices*, he found it fit to request Ellis to write the foreword to it. Ellis felt that the compilation quite definitive and therefore accepted the offer and wrote a juicy foreword to Manfred DeMartino's book, which was published in 1979. The major part of Ellis' foreword was devoted to 50 advantages of masturbation (Ellis, 1979a). At the end of his foreword, he said that he could have easily added 50 more!

Obviously, the main goal of Ellis' writings on masturbation was to encourage and help people enjoy the pleasure of masturbation without being hampered by senseless social and religious taboos. If you are restricted by any religious prohibition on masturbation, Ellis would whole-heartedly urge you to fight against it 'with every pulse of sexuality that you have in your mind and body!'

Homosexuality

Homosexuality is yet another subject to which Ellis had made notable contributions. He had a good deal of experience of offering therapy to sexually disturbed homosexuals. That experience taught him that disturbed homosexuals are not very different from homosexuals as far as their irrational ideas about fidelity, love and intimacy are concerned. What did Ellis think about treating homosexuals? First, he believed that there *should* not be any legal ban on homosexuality. Second, they could be offered treatment only when they are emotionally disturbed about their homosexuality. This means that giving therapy to homosexuals is just like giving therapy to other people (including heterosexuals) who are afflicted with phobias, fixations, obsessions and compulsions. This, in sum, is what originally Ellis believed about homosexuality. In light of Ellis' belief, it becomes understandable why he went to the extent of contributing the article entitled 'A Guide to Rational Homosexuality' to the periodical *Drum: Sex in Perspective* (Ellis, 1964).

With enough experience of treating the disturbed homosexuals to his credit, Ellis (1965b) published the book, *Homosexuality: Its Causes and Cure*. It spells out Ellis's liberal non-judgemental attitudes towards homosexuals. It also shows that Ellis is definitely optimistic about helping emotionally disturbed homosexuals. In fact, a major part of the book is devoted to the application of REBT in treating the disturbed homosexuals.

For example, suppose some homosexuals feel anxious and depressed because they are rejected by a large number of people in their society. In that case, the REBT practitioner will help them identify and challenge the irrational beliefs underlying their unhealthy emotions and replace them by the alternative rational beliefs so that they may only feel concerned and sad about the rejection they experience.

Suppose some homosexuals are eager to practise heterosexuality or at least bisexuality because they want to avoid the social problems created by them being homosexuals. The REBT practitioner will help them switch over to their preferred mode of sexuality. Similarly, if some heterosexuals want to switch over to homosexuality, the REBT practitioner will help them do so. However, it is to be stressed that the REBT practitioner will offer this kind of treatment only to those who wish to adopt a different mode of sexuality.

Ellis admitted that for many years, he believed that males and females who were fixed or exclusive homosexuals could be considered 'neurotics' or even 'borderline psychotics'. This view was re-stated in his book on homosexuality (Ellis, 1965b). However, in the course of time, he agreed with homosexuals who claimed that if they exhibited emotional disturbance, it was because they were condemned by the society in which they lived. Further, they were made to believe that they were worthless because they were homosexuals.

Here, one may ask whether there is any physiological basis for homosexuality. The research done on this subject does not offer any definite answer to this question. Ellis thinks that some confirmed homosexuals might have a slight physiological predisposition to avoid heterosexuals and prefer homosexual relations. Similarly, some heterosexuals might have a slight physiological predisposition to avoid homosexuals and choose heterosexuals. By and large, human beings can change their heterosexuality, homosexuality or bisexuality in spite of their inborn strong tendencies towards their present mode of sexuality.

Therefore, Ellis took a stand that human beings *should* be given freedom to follow the sexual life according to their preferences. There is no question of labelling the homosexuals 'neurotics' or 'borderline psychotics' and attempting to cure them. In short, he fully endorsed the philosophy of Identity House, a counselling centre, in New York City, USA, founded for helping gay and bisexual people. The centre believed that ideally every person *should* be free to choose homosexuality, heterosexuality or bisexuality according to what gives him gratification.

Sexual Abnormality

Ellis did not consider a homosexual as an abnormal person. If so, what did he think about other sexual acts that are usually considered abnormal, perverse or deviant?

This question is to be viewed in light of his views about sexual disturbance in general. It is next to impossible to give a definition of sexual disturbance which would be acceptable to all the experts in the field of sexology, sociology, psychology, etc. However, Ellis explained the meaning of sexual disturbance from the standpoint of REBT. According to him, any emotional disturbance, sexual or non-sexual, is largely a result of three musturbatory ideologies.

1. **Three musturbatory beliefs:** Suppose a man believes in Musturbatory Ideology 1. Then his belief about sexual enjoyment would be, 'I *must* perform well sexually and win the approval of my partner or else I am a *worthless* person'. As a result, he will create anxiety about his sexual performance in his mind. This means that he would be afraid of failing to do sexually well and thereby inviting the disapproval of his partner. He may also restrict

his sexual behaviour to safe acts such as abstinence, masturbation, peeping or sex with children in order to avoid rejection.

Suppose a man believes in Musturbatory Ideology 2. Then his belief about sexual enjoyment would be, 'My partner *must* treat me kindly and help me satisfy myself sexually or else my partner is *worthless* and deserves to be avoided or punished sexually or otherwise'. He will be prone to feel hatred, unlovingness and self-pity. Naturally, he will avoid sex or behave with his partner in a persistently hostile manner.

Finally, suppose a man believes in Musturbatory Ideology 3. Then his demand about sexual enjoyment would be, 'I *must* have easy and quick sexual enjoyment or else it is awful and I *cannot stand* it when I am frustrated or deprived'. Such a man will be handicapped by LFT, hedonism and lack of discipline. In addition, he might foolishly engage in unsafe promiscuity, neglect to take contraceptive precautions and compulsively commit immoral and illegal acts such as rape, sexual assault and seduction of children.

Thus, a man's sexual disturbance is really his emotional disturbance mainly created by his own musturbatory thoughts. His emotional disturbance leads him to the so-called deviant, abnormal or perverse sexual behaviour. There is no reason for condemning and considering him worthless for his supposedly abnormal sexual behaviour. In fact, no sexual act in itself can be labelled abnormal or perverse. Yes, oral and anal sex, fetishistic behaviour, etc. are not abnormal unless one performs any of such acts on an exclusive, obsessive-compulsive, inflexible and self-defeating basis.

Does it mean that acts such as rape and sexual abuse of children, etc. are not perversions? It is true that such acts are immoral, antisocial or criminal. Usually crimes such as robbery, etc. are not called perversions. Hence, there does not seem to be any good reason why only sex offences *should* be scornfully called perversions.

We have seen that the REBT practitioner will offer treatment to homosexuals or heterosexuals who want to overcome their emotional disturbance and want to switch over to more preferred mode of sexuality. Likewise, he will offer help to people who want to overcome their sexual disturbance, that is, their self-defeating thoughts, feelings and behaviour. This means that Ellis' views about the so-called sexual abnormalities including homosexuality are consistently liberal.

2. **Basics of sexual morality:** As regards the many sexual practices of human beings, it is not surprising that people are often perplexed by the problem of normality or abnormality of those practices. They are even more perplexed by the question of the morality or immorality of those practices. In this context, it is worth remembering that even in the 21st century, some devoutly religious people may believe that masturbation is immoral. Scores of people who don't believe in any rigid religious dogma may not be sure whether petting, pre-marital sex, adultery and similar other practices can be considered moral or immoral.

Therefore, it is necessary to reiterate Ellis' concept of general morality, although it is already described in Chapter 7, under the heading 'Sane Morality'. According to Ellis (Phadke, 1999), sexual morality is not any special kind of morality; it is a derivative of general morality. Ellis' concept of general morality is consistent with his philosophy of secular humanism. Humanistic morality is concerned with human goals and not with sub-human goals. It is not unethical to raise and then slaughter some animals for the purpose of making food for human beings. Similarly, human morality is not concerned with the goals of some assumed supernatural gods. Rather, humanistic morality is founded on the nature of man and his desires.

In light of these postulates of secular humanistic ethics, it may be recalled that Ellis offered two fundamental principles of morality. His first principle is *'to thy own self be true'*. This is to be very closely followed by the second principles, *'do not commit any deed that needlessly, definitely and deliberately harms others'*. It is noteworthy that this second principle of morality is just a logical deduction from the first principle.

Though Ellis emphasized the first principle of morality, he alerted not to lose sight on the fact that the second principle of morality recognizes that an individual lives in a society and cannot afford to neglect the interests and rights of others. Ellis also cautioned an individual to look after his short-term as well as his long-term interests and goals. It is unwise to concentrate either only on short-term interests or only on long-term interests. Once this is properly understood, an individual can strive to achieve his personal and social goals without encroaching upon the right of other people to pursue their own interests and goals. Similarly, Ellis' view of morality fully acknowledges the necessity of mutual consent in all human transactions.

3. **Sexual acts:** How did Ellis apply his view about general morality to various sexual acts? Let us take into consideration some sexual practices whose ethical status often becomes a topic of debate.

Masturbation—As this is not a social act, it has nothing to do with morality. An individual who masturbates does not cause any harm to others. Hence, the question of whether masturbation is moral or immoral is irrelevant.

Petting—It is not an immoral social act if it is practised by consenting adults. The act of petting, even when it culminates in orgasm, does no harm to anybody.

Premarital intercourse—If adult and mature people choose to enjoy premarital intercourse with other adult and mature consenting partners, their conduct cannot be called immoral.

Adultery—It is an unethical conduct if it is being committed by a married individual because he breaches the trust which his mate has placed in him. However, if his mate knows that he is an adulterer and permits him to be so, then that is a different issue altogether! If an unmarried individual carries on an affair with a married person, he is not behaving unethically provided that he does not know the mate of his married partner and is not responsible to him in any way.

Sexual assaults and rape—These are definitely immoral acts because they are based on force or coercion. They are attacks on unwilling people and also harm them. It is to be underlined that these acts are immoral not just because they are sexual, but because they are otherwise also immoral. To be more explicit, they are immoral because they involve force and lack of willingly given consent. Moreover, they harm the victims needlessly, definitely and deliberately.

Ellis' view of morality in general and sexual morality in particular was too rebellious to be accepted easily. Yet, they give a glimpse of how he looked at sexual conduct from the standpoint of secular humanism. On the other hand, a man who firmly adheres to some fundamentalist creed may view even oral-genital relations as bestial or ungodly!

Love and Emotional Disturbance

A system of psychotherapy cannot be mainly concerned with normality and/or morality of any love and sex relationship. It addresses itself to the question of causes and cure of emotional disturbance related to love and sex. REBT is no exception to this premise. The emotional disturbance of millions of men and women is associated with their love and sex life. How REBT tries to help such people can be understood better if we first become familiar with Ellis' views about love and sex.

During the last hundreds of years, so much has been said and written about love. Although a lot of that can be dismissed as just poetic or sentimental trash, the fact remains that loving and being loved is exciting, enjoyable and fulfilling experience in life. The place of love in human life is succinctly summarized in Alfred Lord Tennyson's remark that it is better to have loved and lost than never to have loved at all.

From the psychological (and not romantic) point of view, however, love is one among many emotions human beings are capable of experiencing. Like all other emotions, it is based on a strong favourable or positive evaluation of a person one loves. Then it is obvious that if one strongly evaluates a person unfavourably or negatively, one feels the emotion of hatred for that person. It is better to bear in mind that a strong evaluation of a person—either favourable or unfavourable—often tends to be biased or prejudiced.

When two persons love each other, they develop an intense attachment to each other; they seek each other's company; and they tend to be possessive about each other. However, as the emotion of love is based on one's own evaluation of another person, it changes as one's own evaluation of another person changes. In other words, like other emotions, the emotion of love is also subject to birth, growth and decay and even death.

This demystifying way of looking at love may seem to be cold and prosaic. However, it is based on reality. Does it mean that romance and poetry have no place in Ellis' view of life and love? Not at all! On the contrary, he sincerely believed that a rigidly reasoned-out life would become too mechanical, cold, drab and machine like. Romance, poetry and similar other finer things in life have a very legitimate, enjoyable and useful place in life. However, while understanding the causes and cures of emotional disturbance associated with love and sex, we had better take a more dispassionate view of the place of love and sex in life.

Some psychologists believe that love means taking genuine interest in the growth and development of your beloved for the sake of that person and not for the sake of your own interest. No doubt this view sounds noble. However, it does not take into account the fact that many people love another person lightly, promiscuously and without much regard for the growth and development of another person. In that case, will it be correct to say that such people's love for another person is not 'true love'? Yes, if one accepts some arbitrary definition of love. Otherwise, when one loves another person/s in the sense that one feels emotional attachment to that person/s, that love is considered to be real or true just because it exists in the sense one truly feels it.

If a man accepts some arbitrary meanings of true love and sex life, then he tends to live according to those meanings desperately and then may create emotional disturbance in his mind. Because, in the first place, he accepts some unrealistic and irrational ideas or beliefs about love and sex life, and, in the second place, he turns those ideas or beliefs into musturbatory ideologies.

1. **True love:** There are many irrational beliefs which underlie emotional disturbances associated with love and sex, besides the idea that there is something like 'true love'. Table 10.1 lists some of them along with their rational counterparts.

Table 10.1

Irrational and Rational Beliefs of Love

Irrational Beliefs	Rational Beliefs
1. One cannot enjoy sex with another person unless one feels true love for that person.	1. Some people can enjoy sex with another person even if they feel no love for that person.
2. Love is some mysterious force and therefore it cannot be described in a mundane language.	2. Love, like other emotions, is based on one's own evaluation of another person and therefore can be described in a mundane day-to-day language.
3. One can love only one person, at least at a time.	3. One can love many persons even at a time.
4. Love and marriage always go together.	4. One can live with one's married partner without feeling any love for the partner. One can love a person whom one is not married to.
5. If one loves a certain person, one cannot have sexual attachment for some other person/s.	5. Even if one loves a certain person, one can have sexual attachment for some other person/s.
6. When one loves a person, one loves that person all the time.	6. Even when one loves a person, one loves that person intermittently because one has to do many other things in life besides loving the beloved!

Source: Ellis (2003).

Finally, it is necessary to clarify that a man can love another person heterosexually, homosexually or bisexually. Similarly, just as a man can love or develop emotional attachment to human beings, he can also love objects or ideas. Some people live very happily without developing any attachment to any human being.

2. **Use of REBT:** Now it is not difficult to imagine how a man can create unhealthy emotions of anxiety, guilt, depression, jealousy, anger, etc. by subscribing to any or many irrational beliefs and turning them into musturbatory ideologies. While treating such emotionally disturbed people, an REBT practitioner's task is obvious, to help them detect and dispute their musturbatory ideologies with the help of suitable cognitive, emotive and behavioural techniques, and replace them with alternative rational beliefs. Then those people will be free to fulfil their love and sex desires in a sane and sensible manner.

How did Ellis actually work with a client having a sexual problem? Here is a case of Francis presented in Case 10.1.

Case 10.1

Case of Francis

Francis is 30-year-old man. He got married recently. He complains that he ejaculates too quickly while having intercourse with his wife. He feels guilty as he is not able to satisfy his wife. He has also developed self-hatred and experiences the feeling of worthlessness.

Analysis of Case 10.1

Had Ellis been alive, how would he have dealt with Francis? An excerpt of Ellis and Francis' imaginary dialogues is given below.

Ellis: How do you feel when you ejaculate too quickly?

Francis: I feel guilty for coming very quickly—just in 10 or 15 seconds. Then I put myself down for my miserable performance.

Ellis: What do you tell yourself that makes you feel guilty?

Francis: Probably, I tell myself that I *should not* have come so quickly. I *should have* continued the intercourse longer. Then I would have made my wife and myself happy.

Ellis:	Anything more?
Francis:	I tell myself how awful it is that I come so quickly and make both of us feel miserable. This proves that I am a *useless* man.
Ellis:	Do you think what you talk to yourself at such a time is sensible?
Francis:	Yes, because I really want to see that my wife and I enjoy sex longer.
Ellis:	Just because you want to make both of you sexually happy, you *must* last longer when you have intercourse with your wife. Is this what you mean?
Francis:	Yes.
Ellis:	Can you prove your idea that just because both of you want to enjoy sex longer, you *must* last longer?
Frances:	No, I cannot.
Ellis:	Is it really *awful* that you come too quickly?
Francis:	No, but it is quite disappointing.
Ellis:	Good! Which sensible ideas can you tell yourself when you come just in 10 or 15 seconds?
Francis:	I think it is better to tell myself that it is too bad that I have come so quickly, but it is not awful. I don't become a useless man because of the problem I have in my sex life.
Ellis:	If you tell yourself such ideas, how will you feel?
Francis:	Maybe I will feel regret for my poor performance but not guilty. I will then not consider myself a useless person.
Ellis:	Okay. Then you will be left with a practical problem. Can you tell which problem I mean?
Francis:	I think my practical problem will be 'what can I do so that I can last longer while having intercourse with my wife?'

This excerpt is intended to show how the therapist helps the client get rid of unhealthy emotions such as guilt, self-hatred, etc. which complicate his practical problem and adversely affect his problem-solving ability. In order to achieve this goal, the therapist attacks the client's irrational philosophy which, as you would have easily guessed, is 'I *must* have perfect intercourse with my wife or else I am *worthless*'.

The therapist then proceeds to help the client solve his practical problem if possible or to live with his problem gracefully if it is insolvable by maintaining his unconditional self-acceptance.

Of course, the actual therapy sessions with the client do not go as smoothly as this edited and abridged excerpt may seem to suggest. In actual therapy, the therapist uses many cognitive, emotive or behavioural techniques to help the client. The purpose of this excerpt is to show one of the distinguishing characteristics of REBT—helping the client replace his irrational philosophy of life by a rational philosophy of life.

Marriage and Family Problems

Marital discord can have multiple causes. The husband and wife experience dissatisfaction in their relations with each other when they do not get from their partner what they want. Broadly speaking, we may say that their expectations may be about many factors in their lives including economic, occupational and other difficulties.

However, Ellis made a distinction between dissatisfaction and emotional disturbance. When married couples create unhealthy emotions of anger, hostility, depression, guilt, jealousy, etc., in their minds, they find it difficult to overcome their dissatisfactions resulting from many factors in their lives.

An REBT practitioner helps married partners to focus on their own and their partner's musturbatory ideologies underlying their emotional disturbance and then replace them with sensible philosophy of life.

Similarly, when the REBT practitioner is engaged in doing family therapy, he makes a distinction between the dissatisfactions of family members and their emotional disturbance. Family members feel dissatisfied when their expectations of other members of the family are not fulfilled. They become emotionally disturbed when they turn their expectations into demands and then find out that their demands are not met by other members of the family.

The REBT practitioner helps the family members surrender their musturbatory ideologies underlying their unhealthy emotions. Once the family members liberate themselves from their emotional disturbance, they become ready to tackle their practical problems resulting from their living together.

Thus, while offering therapy to married couples or members of a family, the REBT practitioner's main task is to help his clients overcome their emotional problems that compound their practical problems. Only when they have done so, can they be taught to solve their practical problems by learning communication skills, problem-solving techniques, techniques of negotiation, etc.

Emotional Education for Children

One of the most crucial problems married couples face is how to ensure that their children grow without becoming emotionally disturbed or neurotic. In order to consider this question, it is necessary to understand Ellis' views of a neurotic. According to him, anybody who consistently behaves illogically, irrationally, inappropriately and childishly can be called a neurotic. As all children and adults behave in this way, they are, at least to some extent, neurotic. No parents can help their children grow with absolutely no trace of emotional disturbance. However, parents can learn to take some precautions so that eventually their children become largely undisturbed adults.

Of course, if any individual is born with less than average intelligence and therefore behaves stupidly, he cannot be called neurotic as his behaviour is commensurate with his capacity. When an individual is potentially capable of behaving intelligently and yet behaves stupidly, he is to be considered neurotic. This means that neurosis or emotional disturbance is inferred from the gap between an individual's potentiality and actual performance. In other words, his actual performance is below his potentiality which is clouded by his emotional disturbance. Neurosis, therefore, means stupid behaviour of a non-stupid person.

If parents want their children to not perform below their capabilities, they can take some precautions while nurturing them. To guide parents for achieving this objective, Ellis in collaboration with Janet L. Wolfe and Sandra Mosely, wrote the book, *How to Prevent Your Child from becoming a Neurotic Adult*, which was issued in paperback under the title *How to Raise an Emotionally Healthy, Happy, Child* (Ellis, Wolfe & Moseley, 1966). The main thrust of this book is on helping parents achieve two main objectives. First, they have to learn to recognize the irrational beliefs underlying their children's unhealthy emotions and handicapping behaviour. Second, they have to learn to replace those irrational beliefs by rational beliefs. Of course, they have also to give up their irrational beliefs about parenting.

The book is a good REBT-based manual that parents can use to help themselves and their children. Another notable book is *Case Studies in*

REBT with Children and Adolescents (Ellis & Wilde, 2001). This book describes a number of examples of children's emotional problems and throws light on how parents can deal with these problems effectively. Subsequently, some other psychologists also wrote REBT-based manuals for the benefit of parents. Ellis then went one step ahead and decided to experiment with the idea of offering preventive counselling to children in a more systematic and formal manner. In 1970, he founded The Living School in his institute with a view to implementing his programme of emotional education for children.

The Living School

The Living School was a grade school for normal children of age 6–14 and provided education from first to eighth grade. It was a very small school with two classes having around 10 students each. A special feature of the school was that it was primarily meant for children from the middle-class population and from the economically backward strata of society. Hence, about half of them were white middle class and the rest were half Puerto Rican and Black. However, all of them were average children as severely disturbed children were not admitted to the school. The fees were charged according to parents' socio-economic level. Besides, the school offered many scholarships to the children belonging to minority communities.

Curriculum: The academic curriculum of the school was just like other grade schools in New York City. The very purpose of the school was to offer, in addition to the traditional academic education, a novel subject, namely, preventive emotional education. What does emotional education mean? Popularly, it means encouraging children to enjoy themselves, choose what they like to do in various activities in school and outside and express their genuine emotions. Surely, these were worthy objectives. However, they didn't constitute the essence of emotional education as envisaged by The Living School.

The school's concept of preventive education was comprehensive. It was founded on the hypothesis that this additional input would enable children to ensure that in their adulthood, they would deal with their problems of day-to-day living in mature and few self-defeating ways. Needless to say, the principles of REBT formed the basis of this novel educational input (Ellis, 1969).

On this foundation, many stories, short plays, poems, fables and tales were included in the school curriculum. The provision of audio-visual teaching aids was made to teach the curriculum interestingly. Creativity and imagination is the soul of children's cognition. Hence, folktales and fairy tales were also incorporated in the curriculum. Precaution was taken not to inculcate any irrational beliefs in the young minds through them. If famous fairy tales carried such beliefs, instead of barring them entirely, they were adapted with few changes.

One distinct example is Cinderella's fairy tale. In the traditional tale, Cinderella faces some problems and hence approaches the fairy godmother seeking help. The story is fascinating, but it cultivates a number of irrational beliefs in the minds of young children.

First, we need to depend on others to solve our problems as we ourselves are incapable of solving them.

Second, at the time of difficulty, some mysterious power definitely helps us.

Third, our problems get solved instantly like the waving of a magic wand.

While adapting Cinderella's tale, the structure of the original tale was kept untouched but changes were made to instil rational beliefs in young minds. In the new story, it was shown that Cinderella helped herself without taking help from anybody.

Another example was the story of 'Open Boot'. In this story, a brother and sister duo travelled in a boot to take a tour in a fantasyland. In this land, there were talking trees, leaves, flowers, fruits, birds and animals. While conversing with them, the duo gets guidance on healthy and unhealthy emotions.

There were also several poems in the curriculum. Take for example, the poem 'The Little Engine That Could'. In this poem, a little engine chants 'I think I Can! I think I Can!' and climbs a tall mountain. It gives the messages that we *should* never consider ourselves inferior. Believe in yourself. You will be able to achieve high goals by taking small steps.

There were many caselets and playlets which unfolded how we think, talk to ourselves and the consequences of this on our behaviour. There were ample colouring books, boards and playful comics designed on rational principles. Conventional Superman and Batman were replaced by RET Man. With the help of pictures, he was describing various problem-solving methods based on self-reliance.

A variety of workbooks and fun quizzes were also introduced in the curriculum. They consisted of interesting questions to help the children examine their self-talk about themselves, others and about the world. There were riddles describing difficult situations. While solving them, children would find out effective ways on their own. To prevent the expansion of new irrational beliefs, few test series were also accommodated in the curriculum.

Teacher's training: After deciding the curriculum, Ellis had to take a call on whom to devote the responsibility of delivering this curriculum. A special committee had been set up to take a decision on that. It was decided unanimously that the programme of preventive emotional education *should* be implemented by regular school teachers and not by any specially employed psychologist, counsellor or psychotherapist. Of course, the school had employed trained and licensed teachers for teaching the usual academic subjects such as history, geography, mathematics. Additional training was also given to them in the theory and practice of REBT.

The trainee-teachers were given the same kind of training which was given to those who were to become the fellows of the institute. As a result, the trainee-teachers could effectively learn the methods of counselling an individual and also groups of youngsters and adults. In addition, they were given opportunities to benefit from lectures, workshops and other similar programmes that the institute was conducting for the public. Every trainee-teacher was expected to work independently as a counsellor for a group of individuals at least once during the training period. However, the trainee-teacher was expected to acquire this experience under the guidance of a qualified supervisor.

Ultimately, trainee-teachers had to work independently with children in the school. A qualified supervisor would take the role of a counsellor in the group of students and demonstrate the trainee-teacher the technique of handling the problems of students. At the same time, the trainee-teacher was expected to remain alert and observe how the supervisor was tackling the problems of students.

For example, suppose the supervisor of a trainee-teacher was Ellis himself and the trainee-teacher had gone to his office with 6–8 students from her class. Ellis then gave a demonstration of how to counsel students in a group. The trainee-teacher carefully observed the demonstration and learned valuable insights into the counselling process. While counselling, Ellis primarily took the role of a teacher because he believed that offering emotional education to students was basically a process of teaching. Being a good student of his subject, he knew very well the difficulties related to children's thoughts and emotions. He was confident that by using the method of group counselling and some other methods, he could teach students to become more rational and not become victims of self-defeating unhealthy emotions.

Such a demonstration helped the trainee-teacher understand that Ellis did not act merely as a teacher but also discharged his responsibility of teaching students to think in a sensible manner and make life happier. He behaved with students in a friendly manner and played his role in such a way that they not only looked upon him as a loveable person but also as a respectable adult. He felt affinity for them and liked some of their behaviour. When the counselling session was in progress, he encouraged the students when they gave correct answers and showed disappointment when they gave wrong answers. Sometimes, he plodded them to take the risk of doing some unusual activities and to face new experiences. Thus, the trainee-teacher could directly observe how he took the role of a teacher in different ways. When the demonstration was over, Ellis explained to the trainee-teacher the main problems of students he had tried to tackle and how REBT dealt with those problems.

Parents: As the school was launching a novel experiment in the field of education, it was necessary to take into confidence the parents. This was done by informing the parents that giving instructions along with conventional subjects was an integral aspect of school's day-to-day activities.

Parents were told that it was mandatory for them to participate in the monthly workshops organized by the school. In those workshops, problems related to emotional education given to students were discussed. The workshops offered guidance to parents regarding the way they could supplement at home the emotional education their children received in the school. Further, it was suggested to them that they had better acquire at least some basic knowledge of REBT. In order to acquire such knowledge, they were advised to make use of educational materials such books, audiocassettes, etc. brought out by the institute. They were encouraged to profit from the lectures and workshops on REBT which were offered by the institute for the lay people. If parents wanted to solve their own problems, they were free to approach those therapists at the institute who were associated with the school. All such efforts of the school were based on the assumption that to execute its programme of emotional education for the students successfully, parents had to be actively involved in it.

Execution: When all these preparatory steps were successfully executed, the teachers were ready to implement the programme of emotional education in classrooms. How did a teacher actually impart emotional education to students? An example will show how a trained teacher blended the teaching of an academic subject with emotional education. Suppose that, at point A, a student failed in arithmetic and then he felt terribly depressed at point C. At such a time, the teacher brought to that student's attention that his emotion of depression was not created by his failure in arithmetic, but it was caused by the irrational attitude rooted in his mind at point B. That irrational attitude was 'I *must not* have failed in arithmetic; it is terrible that I did fail; and my failure proves that I am a *worthless* and *good for nothing* person'.

Then at point D, the teacher taught him to examine his attitude and see how far it was true. In this way, the teacher motivated him to challenge his own attitude by asking some penetrating questions to himself. These included questions such as 'Where is the evidence to believe that I *must* not have failed in arithmetic? How can my failure prove that I am a *worthless* and *good for nothing* person?'

The teacher did not fail to follow up the process of teaching the student how to dispute his beliefs by giving him some homework assignment. For example, he encouraged the student to deliberately appear for some arithmetic tests. If the student completed the assignment, he might pass those tests, he could learn to feel sad for his failure without condemning himself or putting himself down and feeling depressed. The teacher could go a step further and ask the student to deliberately fail in some undertaking. The idea behind such assignments was that by doing such assignments the student could learn to attack vigorously the irrational attitudes underlying his emotion of depression.

Once the student disputed and destroyed his irrational attitude at point D, he could move to point E. At this point, he would notice two changes in himself. First, a rational attitude towards his failure had firmly replaced his irrational attitude towards his failure. That rational attitude was 'my failure in arithmetic is definitely troublesome and disadvantageous, but there is nothing *terrible* in it. There is no reason to believe that I *must* not have failed in arithmetic. Although, many reasons could be given to support the idea that it would have been better had I not failed, but my failure does not prove that I am a *worthless* and *good for nothing* person. A sensible conclusion from what has happened can be that I have some unfortunate traits. For instance, I may not be quite efficient in arithmetic and to some extent may lack some amount of self-discipline'.

Second, the student would notice that his depression had vanished. He was still feeling sad for failing in arithmetic, but that emotion was helping him to prepare for the next examination with a more determined and relaxed state of mind.

This example shows how the student can be helped to overcome his emotional disturbance by the teacher trained in REBT. But it is necessary to note one point. That is, this example gives only a broad outline of the method the teacher can use to help the student to overcome his emotional disturbance. The process of imparting emotional education to students is neither easy nor very quick, however. First, while imparting this kind of education, the teacher has to take into account the student's age, his level of understanding, the nature of his problem, etc. For example, at point D, it is not easy to teach young students the technique of meticulously disputing their irrational attitudes. Therefore, they are trained to think rationally by using a variety of other methods. For instance, a group of students can be induced to discuss the following two sentences and to learn which is a rational thought and which is an irrational:

1. I want to make excellent progress in my studies because that would be advantageous.
2. I *must* make excellent progress in my studies or else it would mean I am a useless and good for nothing person.

   Challenges: Even if the teacher offered education for emotional hygiene by using a variety of methods to make it easily understandable, two other difficulties arose. First, some students were not willing to learn the fundamental principle of REBT which states that man's emotional disturbance at point C is not caused merely by the events in the external world at point A; it is largely caused by the irrational attitudes rooted in man's mind at point B. Some students thought that events occurring at point A cause emotional disturbance at point C. This notion in their mind can be briefly presented as A $\rightarrow$ C.

Though some students theoretically learnt the formula A $\times$ B = C, they were not willing to overcome their emotional disturbance by using this formula. At such a time, the teacher did not conclude that the resistance shown by the students was a result of their anger towards him or that such students enjoyed remaining emotionally upset. On the contrary, the teacher believed that their resistance was a manifestation of their inborn human tendency to think irrationally. This inborn tendency was also strengthened by their social environment. Thus, their rebellion against rational attitudes and their insistence on behaving in their usual inefficient ways was a result of their pursuit of their short-term gains rather than long-term gains. Similarly, their resistance persisted due to their susceptibility to emotional disturbance. Besides, one more reason for their resistance was that they became slaves of their proneness to think irrationally and self-defeatingly. They also believed how nice it would be if their problems would be solved and the conditions around them were improved magically without requiring any effort on their part!

The teacher knew that while providing emotional education to student, such difficulties did arise and he also knew how to resolve such difficulties. Therefore, the teacher explained to the student which irrational attitude was creating and maintaining resistance in his mind. Similarly, he brought to the attention of the student that his irrational rebellion was likely to bring more disadvantages than advantages to him. Therefore, he encouraged the student to recognize and uproot the irrational attitudes responsible for his rebellion and resistance by persistently working against them.

In short, the trained teacher knew that students would resist his counselling. He also knew that he had better not get upset and give up his efforts at such times. Hence, he persevered in coping with the resistance of students. Naturally, he repeatedly taught the student that if he wanted to free himself from emotional disturbance, he had better uprooted the irrational attitudes from his mind and substitute rational attitudes in their place.

Teaching methods: This was not an easy task. However, teachers in The Living School could observe that even six-year-old first graders benefited from the school's programme of emotional education. Some people may be surprized to know this. They may wonder what meaning the students could understand of the phrase 'Education for Emotional Hygiene' and how they were able to derive benefits from that education. This doubt is certainly understandable and it can be dispelled by stating that the teachers in the school were not offering education for emotional health to students by giving lectures or by using dry, uninteresting methods. On the contrary, the teachers made use of different methods to make the subject interesting and easy to understand. For example, stories, skits, fairy tales and many audio-visual aids were also incorporated in the process of teaching.

Many games were created which could enhance classroom teaching. For example, one game contained picture booklets. Many pictures were depicted in these booklets. In one picture, two children were fighting with each other for a ball. One among them was snatching the ball from another by saying, 'it is my turn now; I will not give it to you'. The reply of another boy was kept blank. It was to be filled up by students by imagining themselves in the place of that boy. They had to report the emotion they would feel in this situation. When each student from the class filled his reply, the booklets were collected and distributed randomly in the class. Children got the opportunity now to know how their classmates think a different reply in same situation. It helped them strengthen the main tenet of REBT, that is, B → C.

Let us see another game. It was called 'Fact Detective'. In this game, teachers wrote on the board a name of any difficult situation. Students were asked to find out the sentences of self-talk. Then, they had to do a work of a detective to search which one of these sentence was independently verifiable and supported by the fact. The student who did this work the best would be declared the winner. The objective of this game was to make the students aware that how many a times we exaggerate or overgeneralize the situation and talk to ourselves unrealistically and to train them in examining their self-talk.

Counselling: When a student was emotionally disturbed, his teacher would counsel him. At such a time, it did not matter whether the student's emotional disturbance was related to his classroom work or his relationship with other students. His teacher was ready to help him even outside his class or outside the school. For example, if the student was upset and behaving dysfunctionally while playing on the school's playground, or when he had gone to a picnic, or to visit a museum, etc., his teacher would direct his attention to his dysfunctional behaviour and goad him to behave in a more healthy and constructive manner.

While imparting emotional education to students as a preventive step, the teacher made use of the technique of group counselling. In such sessions, the teacher showed students, by giving many examples, how at point B they were foolishly indoctrinating themselves with many irrational attitudes. They were also taught how to work persistently to get rid of their deep-rooted irrational attitudes. Thus, students learned that they could take preventive measures to ensure that they would not be emotionally destroyed while facing difficult situations in their future lives. The technique of group counselling was adopted for the purpose of impressing on the students' minds that they could reduce their self-defeating emotional upsets to a greater extent. This, in turn, was supposed to help students make maximum use of their inborn talents to make their lives happy.

The technique of group counselling was used to help students acquire a rational philosophy of life and use it in their present as well as future lives. The sum and substance of this rational philosophy is that no adverse situation needs to be considered awful. One had better unreservedly accept with complete tolerance all human beings, including oneself, with their good and bad characteristics. Even if a man's behaviour is wrong, it is better to remember that he is an imperfect human being, prone to commit mistakes and therefore is not to be devalued as a human being. The message was given to the students that it is good to live one's own life happily, but it is not necessary to be obsessed with the idea that you are a great man and therefore have to work compulsively to prove your greatness. Instead, it is better to behave according to your preferences and goals. While following your path, it is good to understand other human beings and behave with them cordially. While trying to fulfil your own goals by adopting a rational method, you had better keep in mind the well-being and rights of others to fulfil their goals.

The teacher implemented the programme of emotional education by using group counselling with the long-term objective of teaching students a rational and humanistic outlook in such a way that they would leave the school with this outlook deeply embedded in their minds. As the group counselling sessions had this long-term objective, they were not meant only for selected students who showed signs of emotional disturbance. Rather, participation in the group counselling programme was obligatory for all students until leaving the school.

Rational approach: What was the essence of the school's emotional educational programme? In brief, it consisted of teaching the following two beliefs to students.

1. If the conditions around you are not changeable, at least under the present circumstances, then you had better adjust yourself to those circumstances. For example, if the behaviour of your relatives or friends is very troublesome and unfair, it is better to accept that reality and try to cope with it as calmly as possible without unduly upsetting yourself.
2. Eradicate from your mind the belief, 'I *must* get the approval and appreciation from others or else I am a worthless person'. Then you will realize that you don't always have to strictly comply with all the social customs and traditions prevalent in society. You can, at least to some extent, live your life the way you prefer to live.

The school did not believe that every student *must* become a revolutionary as the conditions around us were imperfect and poor in many respects. Nor did the school believe that in order to fulfil one's own hopes and ambitions, every student *must* adopt some practical ways of making the external conditions more favourable to them. On the contrary, the school's policy was that every child had better endeavour to develop his potential in such a way that he would finally be able to take independent decisions with respect to these fundamental issues without becoming needlessly upset. This means that every student would be free to decide for himself under what conditions and to what extent he may adjust to the external world or revolt against it.

If any educational programme or psychotherapeutic system is driving the students to accept a certain political or social ideology, then there is a reason to believe that that political or social ideology is likely to impose too many restrictions on the students' thinking and thereby limit their freedom of choice. As REBT is based on humanistic and liberal principles of living one's life, the institute carefully avoided giving any rigidly controlled education to its students.

Outcome: What was the outcome of the institute's experiment of providing prophylactic mental health education to children by founding its own private school? The institute expected that students who would join The Living School in the first grade and leave it after completing the eighth grade would be emotionally less disturbed than other students in America who would complete their primary education in other schools. However, the school did not unrealistically expect that its students would be completely free from self-defeating emotions, such as, anxiety, depression and hostility, and that their behaviour would show no deficiencies. Of course, the school did expect that the self-defeating emotions of its students would be improved to a greater extent. Yet, the school obviously did not expect that its students would become angels in their future lives. After all, the students were human beings and, like all human beings, would live their lives as imperfect and fallible beings.

Keeping in mind the school's modest expectations, one may say that it was successful in many aspects, although it became a liability for the institute financially. Only due to this reason, the institute closed the school in 1975. During its five years of existence, the school incurred a loss of one million dollars.

However, the institute's novel experiment of providing preventive emotional education for students showed that if teachers teaching conventional subjects could be trained in REBT, they would effectively counsel normal children aged 6–14.

The school was adjudged a success by its directors. Parents were appreciative of their children's improved emotional health. Such positive effects were more readily seen in children belonging to older age groups. Even some six-year-old students in the first grade were also benefited by the emotional education received in the school. After many years, when some students of the school happened to meet Ellis, they specifically told him that they were continuing to derive benefit of the emotional education they had received in the school.

No systematic follow-up studies were conducted by the school to assess the results of its emotional education programme due to many reasons. For instance, the total number of the students in the school was too small. Many parents wanted to send their children to bigger schools. In bigger schools, students could get more facilities for learning music, varied games and physical exercises. Therefore, some students used to leave the school within 2–3 years. As a result, the school could not do any systematic research to assess the effect of emotional education on its students.

Yet, the school gave rise to two creditable outcomes. First, Gerald and Eyman (1980), who were among the teachers in the school, wrote a book showing how they used REBT in the classroom. Besides, the school produced other materials that could be used to offer emotional education to students. The second interesting outcome was that the school became a source of inspiration to those who wanted to impart preventive education or mental hygiene to students. For example, a school in Connecticut introduced REBT into its curriculum with the help of the Albert Ellis Institute. The teachers in the school participated in a five-day primary certificate practicum given by the institute. Similarly, many teachers, principals and school counsellors participated in the institute's practicum and some of them adapted the institute's materials and used them in their work with students.

Thus, one can justifiably conclude that The Living School was an innovative and fruitful experiment in education.

Alcoholism and Substance Abuse

Alcoholics and substance abusers are common practically in any country. Some of them are addicted to various kinds of alcoholic drinks, whereas some are addicted to different narcotic substances. Incidentally, people get addicted not only to things that they can eat and drink but also various other activities such as gambling. Addiction is widespread phenomenon. In regards to alcoholism, it can be caused by several factors. Some of the commonly discussed reasons of addiction to alcohol or narcotic substances are discuss in the succeeding sections.

Causes of Addiction to Alcoholism

Disease: Why do people get addicted to alcohol or narcotic substances? One frequently given answer to this question is that a man drinks excessively because he is afflicted with the disease of addiction. His disease is responsible for the fact that he drinks intemperately and goes into a state of stupor.

In the vast literature of alcoholism, one comes across a lot of discussion about whether or not addiction to alcohol is a disease. However, it is not necessary to go into details of this question. Suffice to say that whether a man's addiction is a disease or it is his voluntarily accepted slavery, there is only one excellent remedy for it. That remedy is to stop consuming alcohol or other narcotic substances. Suppose somebody's addiction is his disease and therefore he does not give up drinking, his health will then deteriorate even more. On the contrary, suppose another man's addiction to alcohol is not a disease but he voluntarily accepted slavery of alcohol and does not liberate himself from his slavery, then the problems that are created by his unbridled drinking, which are already wrecking him, will be further aggravated. Hence, the best thing he too can do is stop drinking.

Believing that an addiction is a disease has one advantage. It creates the possibility of depending on medical treatment for curing that disease. The theory that a man's addiction is a disease is found attractive to a confirmed drunkard. Because, accepting this theory, he can adopt a defensive posture for freeing himself from the responsibility of any small or big crime. He may say, 'what can I do? When I committed that particular crime, I was in a state of intoxication. My addiction to alcohol is a kind of disease'.

A drunkard who has not committed any crime can also take a different advantage of this theory. He can easily say, 'as the case of my drinking is some kind of a disease which has afflicted me, I can't help drinking. In fact, I drink against my wish. What can I do? The disease which has afflicted me drives me to the bar and forces me to drink non-stop!' In this way, an addict can throw his responsibility overboard. Naturally, he does not blame himself. Therefore, the question of making himself overwhelmed by his guilt does not arise at all.

Biological factors: A man can resort to some other theories too for shirking his responsibility. One of those theories states that some people get attracted to alcohol because of some biological factors within them. As a matter of fact, taking into consideration the conclusions of scientists in this respect, we can say that a man's biological constitution may contribute to his addiction to some extent. It does not mean that a man endowed with a specific genetic inheritance has no alternative but to get himself addicted to alcohol. With the use of his rationality, he is ultimately capable of prevailing over this rather unfortunate, though inborn inheritance, by making efforts.

Somebody is all set to justify his addiction to alcohol by enlisting the support of his hereditary endowment. When he does that, not only is he able to defend his hankering after alcohol but also free himself from the necessity of shouldering the responsibility for his addictive behaviour. Consequently, he does not upset himself by blaming himself and feeling guilty.

Environment: There is one more theory that comes handy to an addict for denying the responsibility for his addiction. According to this theory, the cause of a man's addiction can be found in his family and surrounding situation. If a man is forced to live in an impoverished environment from his childhood, he is driven by that environment to addiction. In fact, the cause of man's addiction is his entire family's addiction to alcohol! Some people find this interpretation of their addiction to alcohol very attractive because, by resorting to it, they think that their addiction is caused by their poor and unhealthy environment, childhood experiences, addicted family members, etc. and thereby they absolve themselves of their responsibility for their addiction. Moreover, by justifying their addiction in this manner, they feel free to continue their addiction in the future.

The last road which is available to a man for passing on the responsibility for his addiction to external factors and freeing himself from the responsibility is to adopt the stance, 'I am helpless; alcohol and other narcotic substances have such a strange power that I am attracted to them unknowingly against my wish'.

It cannot be denied that this theory, so useful in vindicating one's addiction, is interesting. An addict never seems to wonder if there is some strange power in narcotic substances that pulls a man towards them, how is that not all people are pulled in the same way. In a nutshell, the only advantage of this theory is that by resorting to it, an addict is able to avoid responsibility for his bad habit and gets a license to continue his addiction. Instead of saying that he has embraced his addiction, he says that his addiction has embraced him and has held him in the clutches!

Mental slavery: Then what are the causes of man's addiction to alcohol and narcotic substances? The answer to this question is that there are many complex reasons why some people become slaves of certain substances whereas others don't accept the slavery of substances that can be eaten, drunk, smoked or taken into the body through veins or turn to addictions such as gambling.

As regards to drinking, it may be said that some people are attracted to alcohol because of some biological factors in them. Sometimes newspapers, periodicals and other media imply that some people give themselves up to drinking owing to their genes! Their genes compel them as it were to surrender themselves to alcohol. Propagation of such an idea cannot be considered a sign of responsibility. Scientists, however, rarely make such irresponsible statements. According to them, to some extent, a man's genetic make-up contributes to his temptation of alcohol. Although some biological factors in a man somewhat help him get stimulated to drink, it does not mean that a man who drinks has no other alternative but to drink. In reality, he is free to use his ability to think and take his own decisions.

Eventually, more research in the future can probably reveal the specific contribution made by biological factors to a man's compulsive drinking. Nobody can deny that in the light of future scientific progress in this field, new techniques of overcoming alcohol dependence can possibly become available. At present, it is evident that some attitudes of a man are largely responsible for his slavery to alcoholic substances or addiction to gambling. As he is capable of taking decisions, he has voluntarily accepted the mental slavery to addictions. Nothing has thrust that slavery upon him. He can choose to turn his back on the very substance of which he has become a slave.

Essentially, a man's addiction is an attitude and a way of thinking arising out of that attitude. Or, to put in other words, the mental component of addiction includes a man's philosophy of life. Suppose, a man likes to eat sweets, and therefore relishes eating them and enjoys the pleasure he cherishes. If after some time he is afflicted with diabetes and is advised by his doctor to stop eating sweet substances or at least to reduce their proportion in his meals, what will he do? If his liking for sweet substances is only that, that is, liking, he will not find it very difficult to implement his doctor's advice. On the contrary, if he has convinced himself that no matter what happens, a certain amount of sweet substance has to be included in his daily food intake, not only will he find it difficult but also absolutely impossible to implement his doctor's advice.

If he has turned his liking for sweet substances into an absolute necessity, how can he tolerate the idea of eliminating or reducing the sweet substances from his daily intake of food? Now he doesn't only like to consume sweet substances but his fondness for sweet substances has also become his addiction. By surrendering himself to sweet substances, he has made himself a slave of them. If he does not heed to his doctor's advice and continue to devour sweet substances as before, the mental side of his behaviour of eating is his faulty philosophy: 'I *must* get the things I like and which I find alluring'.

Common Methods to Liberate from Addiction

There are many other methods available to liberate people from their addictions. Besides, of course, the medical treatment which is beyond the scope of this book.

Self-help: The first and perhaps the oldest method is self-help! A man can resolve to give up his addiction and implement his resolve. An outstanding example is the famous American playwright Eugene O'Neill. When he was at the zenith of his literary career, he was so addicted to alcohol that he was on the verge of death. Even then, one day, he gave up the slavery of alcohol. Afterwards, he made a substantial contribution to literature and became more famous.

Oath: Some people adopt yet another path for liberating themselves from their addictions. That path is to bid goodbye to your self-destructive addiction by taking an oath that you would not go back to your addiction for the sake of God, your parents, your children or some other beloved persons.

Books: Yet another method adopted by some addicts is to study a book or some other literature. A number of people have gotten rid of their slavery of bad habits with the help of audiocassettes, television programme, etc.

Alcoholic anonymous: A very well-known method of helping people to liberate themselves from addictions (especially alcoholism) is developed by the internationally renowned organization called Alcoholics Anonymous (AA). Millions of people from all over the world participate in the programmes conducted by this organization and at least thousands of them get rid of their addictions.

Yet, some people are not inclined to take advantage of the opportunities offered by AA for many reasons. One of those reasons is that some people are not interested in the programmes of AA or similar other organizations because their views are sceptical. Or, it can be said that although such people may not be atheists or agnostics, they are not inclined to pray for the mercy of God or some other supernatural or spiritual power for breaking their habit of drinking.

If a drunkard says that he is not inclined to join AA or similar other organizations because of reasons like those stated here, the champions of AA would try to convince him that it is absolutely wrong to say that in the programmes of AA, a man is required to pray for the mercy of God or some other supernatural or spiritual power. He will also be told that because AA is based on an all-inclusive, liberal and non-demanding principle, people holding any viewpoint can definitely join it. Moreover, the concept of supernatural or the spiritual inherent in the programmes of AA is so comprehensive that agnostics or even atheists can be extremely benefited by those programmes.

In order to strengthen this argument, the supporters of AA can offer some proof to people who hold sceptical views. They try to prove their point by arguing that AA conducts some special programmes for agnostics. However, some of the people who participate in such special programmes realize that AA gives a step-motherly treatment to such programmes and also a secondary position.

Even if we set aside these experiences of some people, we can understand the attitude of AA towards agnostics from a chapter in *The Big Book* (Alcoholics Anonymous, 2013) which gives a detailed account of the doctrine of AA. In that chapter, the agnostics are derided as if only with the intention of impressing on the reader's mind, the importance of faith in God or some supernatural power.

There is a booklet which gives information about AA. The caricature of a non-believer depicted on the front cover of the booklet entitled *AA: An Interpretation for the Non-believers* (Weinberg, 1975) is worth observing carefully. The central theme of the booklet is that the non-believer's eyes are opened; he realizes his mistake and thereafter begins to live his life happily. Therefore, some people who are familiar with this booklet as well as AA's 12-step programme find it very difficult to accept the idea that AA is not a religious or spiritual organization.

Alternative paths: Whether AA is consistent with secularism or not, the fact remains that many alternative paths to liberation from addictions are available to non-believers. For example, Organization for Sobriety, Women for Sobriety, and Men for Sobriety are some of the organizations that offer de-addiction programmes that do not bother to seek support of spiritual concepts. However, it cannot be overemphasized that it would be dogmatic to claim that among the many ways which are available to a man for liberating himself from addictions, only one particular way is the best and therefore it would be useful to all addicts equally. Obviously, not all people are alike; not all addicts have the same addictions; and only one particular way is neither acceptable nor useful to all people.

REBT Approach

By now, you would have guessed Ellis' approach to diagnosis and treatment of alcoholism. Broadly speaking, Ellis' approach to addictions consists of helping the addict to detect and destroy his faulty philosophy of life. Obviously, it is based on REBT. Its first detailed presentation is to be found in a book titled *Rational Emotive Therapy with Alcoholics and Substance Abusers* (Ellis et al., 1988). Subsequently, he authored another book, *When AA Doesn't Work for You: Rational Steps to Quitting Alcohol*, with Emmett Velten (Ellis & Velten, 1992). Both the books focus on disputing the irrational philosophy of addicts and replacing it with rational philosophy.

There is another book called *The Small Book: A Revolutionary Alternative for Overcoming Alcohol and Drug Dependence* written by Jack Trimpey (1992) who obtained the degree of MSW in 1969 from Wayne State University. In addition, he received extensive post-graduate training in REBT at the Albert Ellis Institute. Then, in the late 1980s, he founded the organization called, Rational Recovery Systems in California. The organization began to offer an REBT-based de-addiction programme.

In his introduction to Jack Trimpey's book, Ellis says that it is one of the very best books available for alcoholics and substance abusers. One of the most enlightening part of Jack Trimpey's book is that it offers 15 irrational beliefs of alcoholism. Those beliefs are adaptations of irrational beliefs frequently encountered in the writings of Ellis. Further, the book also gives rational counterparts of those beliefs. In other words, Jack Trimpey presents the irrational philosophy of addicts and its rational counterpart. The 15 irrational beliefs of addicts and their 15 counterparts are as follows (the rational counterparts are printed in italics and presented in parentheses):

1. Controlling the enormous attraction that I feel for alcohol or similar other narcotic substances is beyond my capacity. As I am so helpless, powerless and impotent, I am not responsible for what I put into my mouth, nose or veins.

   (*I am capable of exercising control over my hands, mouth and some other limbs of my body to a large extent. Therefore, I alone am responsible for what substance I put into my mouth, nose or veins.*)

2. I *must* give up my addiction in order to feel that I am a worthwhile person.

   (*As I believe that I am at least valuable to myself, I have decided to give up my addiction and live a good life.*)

3. As my pain as well as my intense craving for a substance such as alcohol is impossible to control, it is necessary that I relieve my suffering by consuming that kind of substance.

(*If I want to overcome my addiction and live a sober life, at least to some extent, it is necessary, inevitable and safe to tolerate some discomfort.*)

4. The emotions I experience are thrust upon me by some people or specific circumstances; therefore, it is impossible to control those emotions.

   (*Emotions I experience are generated by my thoughts. Therefore, I am capable of exercising a great deal of control over my unhappiness and emotional excitement.*)

5. If even adults crave for approval, respect and love of other people, then it is absolutely necessary that they get those things.

   (*It is not necessary for adults to get the desired approval, respect and love of other people. If other people disapprove of me, or are displeased with me, it only reveals their opinion about my worth. I can either gullibly agree with their opinion or thoughtfully differ from it. Whatever it may be, I always choose to love myself. I feel more pleasant when I love myself rather than when I hate myself. I believe that as regards choosing to love myself, only my decision is final.*)

6. As I have committed some wrong acts, behaved insultingly with some people and harmed somebody, I *must* blame myself for such immoral behaviour, condemn myself and consider myself guilty and worthless.

   (*Although it is understandable that I feel regret, sorrow and remorse because I acted wrongly after I consumed a narcotic substance, it is not necessary to brand myself as 'a worthless person'. Like all human beings, I am also a uniquely fallible person.*)

7. People *must* not behave wrongly. If they behave wrongly, they *should* be blamed, condemned and punished.

   (*Everybody commits mistakes. Therefore, it is meaningless to condemn other people because they behave imperfectly and wrongly. When I say other people don't behave as expected, it means that I am shirking to accept reality! If I condemn others for their mistakes, I will apply the same rule to my behaviour and consider myself guilty and worthless.*)

8. In order to consider myself a worthwhile person, I *must* be efficient, flawless, intelligent and victorious in all respects. If I discontinue consuming some narcotic substance and start consuming it again after some time or if I fail in any similar way, it will be like

supplying evidence to prove what I have always suspected I am an imperfect, inferior and worthless person.

(*It is more important to do something rather than to do it perfectly. To start doing a task is the first step towards becoming successful. I can easily accept myself by believing that although I am a fallible human being, I am a valuable person to myself. I don't become a 'successful man' even if I am successful in some work. Similarly, even if I am unsuccessful in any work, I don't become an 'unsuccessful man'.*)

9. It is awful if events in the environment around me don't happen as I expect them to happen.

(*What does the word 'awful' imply? It implies that a situation around me is completely unfortunate and more than 100 per cent bad. However, the situation is not probably so bad. Similarly, it is not necessary to believe that for me to give up my addiction and live my life happily, peacefully and without getting upset, there has to be a specific situation around me. Even though I may not be able to change the situation around me or cannot bring it under my control, I can accept any calamity, even death if inevitable!*)

10. The events in my past life are mainly responsible for my present emotions and behaviour.

(*The emotions that I am experiencing today are caused by the thoughts I think today. My present behaviour is largely motivated by my current emotions. In the past, I might have learnt to make myself miserable, but today I can change my attitudes and opinions about the unhappiness, calamities, disappointments and losses in the past.*)

11. I am now liberated from my addiction. Therefore, I *must* not even touch narcotic substances, no matter what. Even if I consume such a substance once, I will destroy myself.

(*Gradually, as days pass, I will be fully convinced that consuming narcotic substances is foolish. I will be able to nicely experience how greatly benefited I am by sobriety. In case I do consume a narcotic substance at some time, no awful calamity will befall me immediately. I will, for the sake of my well-being, return to the path of sobriety shortly, without succumbing to the feeling of guilt.*)

12. As I am a slave of narcotic substances, I *must* depend on something or someone more powerful than me.

(*Dependence is my main problem! It would be advantageous to me to start shouldering the responsibility of thinking and acting independently. In fact, I am not an 'addicted person'. I happen to be a man who has accepted some of the attitudes knowingly or unknowingly which aid and abet addictions.*)

13. In the past, my life had become wretched due to my addiction. Therefore, in the future also that addiction will pursue me for an indefinite period of time and frequently make my life wretched.

(*I will enjoy living my life free of addictions. As there are many other things in life which are worth doing besides continuously struggling to remain sober, I will gradually turn my back on my past addiction. Similarly, I will be absorbed in doing only such enjoyable things which are in no way related to my past addiction.*)

14. In order to feel that I am a good man, solicitous about the welfare of others, I *must* feel perturbed by the problems which others face and help them solve their problems.

(*Helping others is not a royal road to proving my moral superiority; and my own perturbation will interfere with my work of helping others.*)

15. Problems of life have flawless and perfect solutions. If I don't find out such solutions, I will be condemned to a life of perennial uncertainty, turmoil and anxiety.

(*Uncertainty is the spice of life and it is foolish to go on finding out perfect solutions to all problems of life. On the contrary, I shall look at life as an enjoyable and advantageous experiment and concentrate on doing things which I like and are conducive to my growth.*)

A careful study of irrational beliefs of addicts will reveal that Jack Trimpey has ingeniously restated Ellis' delineation of irrational beliefs underlying emotional disturbance in such a way that they specifically express the irrational beliefs of addicts. Of course, even those specific irrational beliefs can be categorized into Ellis' three musturbatory ideologies—towards oneself, towards other and towards the external conditions.

Now, it is not difficult to understand how the REBT practitioner helps addicts give up their addictions. Evidently, first, he helps them detect, dispute and demolish the irrational beliefs underlying their addictive behaviour. Second, he helps them inculcate alternative rational beliefs. In order to achieve these goals, the REBT practitioner makes judicious use of cognitive, emotive and behavioural methods.

Here, an explanation is in order. As previously mentioned, Jack Trimpey had received training in REBT at the Albert Ellis Institute. The main emphasis of his book (Trimpey, 1992) is on showing how REBT can be useful for overcoming alcohol and drug dependence. Subsequently, he evolved his own system of helping alcoholics and substance abusers which was totally different from REBT. One of the good sources of information about his system of treatment is his book, *Rational Recovery: The New Cure for Substance Addiction* (Trimpey, 1996). Even in this book, he recommends REBT as one of the alternatives to religio-spiritual teachings and lifestyle of AA.

Yet, the fact remains that irrational beliefs of alcoholism, as presented in Jack Trimpey's book (Trimpey, 1992), are very useful in understanding Ellis's approach to alcoholism and substance abuse.

Getting Older Gracefully

Many people are afraid of old age. They believe that old age is the worst period of life. According to them, old age means impairment of physical and mental abilities, financial problems, dependence on others, rejection by youngsters, illness and finally death. Consequently, such people may just refuse to accept the fact that they are gradually ageing. They then pretend to be young and try to talk, feel and act like young people. Their childish efforts to hide their age from others and themselves make them laughable or even ridiculous in the eyes of others and perhaps in their own eyes too! Hence, they feel more miserable.

Can such people learn to look at the process of ageing in a more constructive and healthy way? Indeed, they can. A number of popular books provide guidance to *old people* on how they can live productively and happily in old age. How can REBT help *old people* stop whining about their lot and live and thrive energetically? That is exactly what Ellis shows in the book, *Optimal Aging*, written with Emmett Velten (Ellis & Velten, 1998). Written in a witty style, the book offers a philosophy of life that can enable *old people* enjoy life even better than they might have enjoyed in their youth! Incidentally, Ellis' one audiocassette on this subject is called *How to Age With Style* (Ellis, 1992).

Of course, Ellis does not mean to say that old age has no hassles. As he preaches a realistic and rational philosophy of life, he will be the last person to advocate any kind of pollyannaism. On the contrary, he shows how one can tackle the hassles of old age by using one's intelligence and knowledge. In fact, one can learn to reduce the handicaps and inconveniences of old age by not being unduly upset about them. Hence, his approach is based on the full acceptance of the fact that the process of getting older involves many problems—some soluble, some partly soluble and some insoluble. The wisdom lies in trying to solve the problems which are soluble and partly soluble, and to gracefully accept the insoluble problems and live with them, rather than continuously moaning and screaming about them.

You may think that this approach of Ellis is quite humdrum and there is nothing new about it. If you think so, you are partly right because Ellis does not offer any radically new goals to *old people*. However, the methods he recommends for achieving those goals are singular.

If *old people* know that they had better stop bemoaning about their age and begin to live enthusiastically and creatively, why do many of them not act according to their wisdom? One possible reason for their failure to live happily is that their irrational attitudes make them depressed and inactive. Ellis' approach precisely shows them how to recognize their irrational and immobilizing beliefs and replace them with rational and motivating beliefs.

Ageism

As the first step towards following the path to happy living, Ellis cautions *old people* that ageism is quite common in almost any society. Ageism means prejudice against *old people*. As a matter of fact, it is not an exaggeration to say that many *old people* are afraid of old age because they know that prejudice against old age is widespread.

Unfortunately, some *old people* are prejudiced against themselves and other *old people*. The first thing *old people* can do is to fight the very concept of ageism. The most effective way to do this is to stop considering themselves *old people* and begin to consider themselves *older people*. What is the reason for preferring the word 'older'? The simple answer Ellis gives to this question is that strictly speaking no group of people can be called '*old people*'. The age of any human being is always growing from the minute he is born until he breaths his last. Every second a man is getting older. Therefore, the concept of old age is misleading, whereas the concept of '*older people*' is realistic. Once a man starts considering himself an *older man*, he bridges the so-called gap between young people and *old people*.

It may seem that it is unnecessary to make such a fuss about ageism. However, it is not correct to treat ageism as a trifle. Ageism implies an idea that human worth depends on a man's age. It gives the impression that young people are worthwhile, whereas *old people* are worthless. It also goads people to hide the natural biological changes that accompany advancing age. As one can easily infer, this prevents *old people* from accepting themselves unconditionally.

Granted that if *old people* call themselves *older people*, they will fight ageism instead of explicitly or implicitly succumbing to it and emulating younger people. But how does Ellis help them live happily? First, he encourages them to cherish the slogan: *carpe diem* (seize the day). This means that they *must* actively pursue happiness here and now, and at this moment. Don't wait for an auspicious day to start living happily. Second, he offers one of the most important principles of REBT to them. Obviously, the message states that 'one feels the way one thinks'. Third, he offers '20 rules' for growing older happily and gracefully. Let us, therefore, understand the 10 most important of those 20 rules.

Rules for Growing Older Happily and Gracefully

Rule No. 1: *Face reality*. It is good for you to accept the fact that there are good, bad and indifferent aspects of ageing. Suppose you go for a medical check-up and are diagnosed with diabetes or some other disease/s. In that case, it is irrational to deny or neglect the reality about your health and go on living life without doing anything about it. On the contrary, it is rational, that is, self-helping to accept that reality and follow the doctor's advice. Surely, life is tough with ill health because it can become tougher by not accepting your ill health. This may seem too obvious to be mentioned. It is amazing how often *older people* aggravate their problems—related or unrelated to their health—by just refusing to face facts.

Rule No. 2: *Take action*. If you want to be happy, start taking some active steps to make yourself happy. The world does not owe you happiness. Don't believe that other people are terribly busy in finding out ways to make you happy. Rely on self-help! Even if you want to cultivate a simple hobby, get up and begin to do something about your goal. Once you actively pursue your goal, you increase the chances of achieving it.

Similarly, if you accept the fact that you have diabetes and want to get adequate medical treatment for it, push yourself to go to some medical specialist and rigorously follow his advice. Don't delay; inaction in such matters can be dangerous, or even fatal!

Why do many people fail to cultivate even a simple hobby or seek and follow the advice of a medical specialist? They are great devotees of the philosophy of LFT. REBT shows them how they can dispute that handicapping philosophy and begin to pursue their goals actively.

Rule No. 3: *Create yourself.* Accept the fact that you cannot change some aspects of the conditions under which you live. You cannot even change your own age! Your age and some conditions are activating events (As) in your life. However, you can learn to change your beliefs (Bs) about them. You can then create more desirable emotional consequences (Cs) in your mind which will motivate you to modify the changeable conditions around you, and then do what you want to do. You can learn to hold rational beliefs about ageing so that you can feel enthusiastic about your goals and also direct your energies towards their fulfilment. If you continue to cling to irrational beliefs about ageing, you will create unhealthy emotions in your mind and dissipate your energy.

Rule No. 4: *Accept responsibility.* Take care to focus on the main powerful message of the $A \times B = C$ theory. The message is that no matter how adverse the conditions under which you live are, you have enough freedom to choose what to think about them. It is not correct to yield to the idea that you are doomed to be a helpless puppet controlled by the conditions around you. On the contrary, you have the capacity to choose your own way of responding to the circumstances around you.

Suppose you have acquired some unhygienic habits of eating, drinking, etc. and you want to give up those habits. Stop blaming your parents, relatives, friends, other people, or the conditions under which you spent your childhood for forcing you to acquire those habits. None of those factors forced you to learn and retain those habits. Maybe, those factors contributed to your acquisition of those habits, but only you decided to act as per the stimulation provided by those factors. Accept the fact that you were responsible for learning and maintaining those habits. You will then be able to re-think and develop rational attitudes towards them. This change in your beliefs will help you to give up those habits on your own. It will be nice if you get help from others when you are working at changing your habits. However, you can bring about a change in yourself by your own efforts.

Rule No. 5: *Do it now.* You might have nurtured a dream of how to live your life after retiring from your service or business. After your actual retirement, you might not have done anything to materialize your dream. In fact, your dream might have evaporated. Now you may be feeling depressed for having done practically nothing to achieve your dream!

Why have you created such a situation in your life? One reason can be that you have become a slave of the belief that you are incapable to pursue your fond goal of living happily because your childhood experiences moulded your personality so strongly that now you cannot do anything new. You might have even gullibly accepted the idea that a man's personality is shaped in the first five or six years of his life and he then is left with little freedom to make any changes in himself. Perhaps, you have learned this idea even from a psychotherapist or a book authored by a psychiatrist.

On the contrary, Ellis' $A \times B = C$ theory asserts that a man's childhood experiences do not directly mould his personality. His own interpretation and evaluation of his childhood experiences influence his personality. He can choose to examine, challenge and give up the ideas that he might have accepted in his childhood (or even adulthood).

If you decide to pursue your goals after retiring from your service or business, your childhood and other experience will have no power to stop you. Only you have the power to pursue your goals or prevent you from realizing your dreams. Once you accept this idea, you will not find it difficult to start taking steps to actualize your dreams immediately.

Rule No. 6: *You can't change the past.* No matter how much you cry over the unpleasant events in your past life, they are gone and over! Nothing can change them. Merely brooding over the gruesome events in your past life will neither change them nor help you follow some creative pursuits. On the contrary, continuously recalling the bad events of your past makes you pessimistic about your present and future life.

Surely, you understand that the past cannot be changed and weeping and wailing over it would make your present and future life miserable. What do you do then? You may try to solve the problem by becoming a great devotee of positive thinking. You may begin to tell yourself that 'day by day, in every way, I am getting better and better'. It is not a bad solution because at least it distracts you from brooding over unhappy events of your past. It seems to suggest that you *must* succeed and be approved by others or else you are no good. As Ellis says, positive thinking is more practical than philosophical. If you tell yourself 'I can work towards my goals', you will be motivated to work for the achievement of goals. However, if you tell yourself 'even if I don't do well, I am determined only to rate my performance and never to condemn myself', your method can be considered philosophical.

Perhaps, you may think, as you grow older, you had better develop serenity or desirelessness when you face obstacles in life. This approach is likely to defeat your goal of living happily. REBT neither asks you just to think positively nor does it advise you to develop a detached or serene life. It believes that healthy negative emotions, such as, concern, sadness, grief, disappointment, annoyance and frustration, are good because they may inspire you to overcome the obstacles in your path to happiness. Of course, REBT advises you to get rid of unhealthy emotions, such as, anxiety or panic, depression, guilt, shame and embarrassment, rage, anger, hatred and revenge, since these emotions obstruct your path to happiness.

Although you cannot change the past, experiencing healthy negative emotions about the past is good, if they motivate you to learn from your past and work for creating happiness in your present and future life.

Rule No. 7: *Accept and forgive yourself unconditionally.* Theoretically, you will have no difficulty in understanding the idea that it is better to forget the unpleasant events in your past because they cannot be changed or wiped out by positive thinking. You may find it difficult to forget many unfortunate events in your past life. One reason for your continuing to dwell on the past (in spite of your determination not to do so) may be that you believe you *should not* have committed certain mistakes or you *should not* have behaved harshly with the people you love. In fact, you may spend a lot of time in digging up the unpleasant events in your life that make you feel ashamed of yourself. Then, you may wallow in self-pity, guilt or even self-hatred. You may even try to atone your past mistakes or sins! Yet, you don't stop your brooding over the ghastly memories of the past. That is why you find it so difficult to act on the precept, 'forget the past'.

If you are really suffering because disturbing memories of the past haunt you, REBT can help you overcome the bad influence of the past and live in the present and for future. It teaches you to accept yourself in spite of your mistakes, that is, unconditionally. Indeed, Ellis' concept of USA will show you how to acknowledge your own mistakes and even regret them without berating yourself, that is, your totality. The lesson to learn is that you are not equal to your past, present or future mistakes. You are a unique, living human being who commits mistakes. You commit mistakes because you are a fallible human being—neither devil nor god. If you unconditionally accept yourself as a fallible human being, you will be able to forgive and release yourself from the chains of your disturbing memories and concentrate on enjoying the remaining life.

Rule No. 8: *Get absorbed in some vital interest.* You are more likely to feel happy and healthy when you are involved in something outside yourself. If you are handicapped by some ailments and disabilities, it is all the more useful to be absorbed in pursuing a goal that you find interesting. You can get involved in ideas, projects or people. Who can say what you would like to do? Explore different areas of activity and go on experimenting with some of them with a view to discovering a goal that can keep you absorbed for a fairly long period. Maybe you decide that you can get yourself involved in more than one goal. If you whole-heartedly pursue your goal, you will enjoy the process of working towards its realization. When you devote yourself single-mindedly to the achievement of your goal, you will stop thinking irrationally. Also, you bear up unavoidable troubles of life with relative ease.

All in all, you have a good chance of growing older gracefully if you get involved in some vital interest. Of course, this is not a new idea. REBT warns you not to succumb to the belief that you *must* be successful in materializing your dream. By all means, work at fulfilling your dream, but don't conclude that you are a worthless person if you fail to realize your dream. If you take heed to this warning, you will enjoy the process of working towards your cherished goal without feeling desperate about succeeding in it. Or, to borrow the words of Ellis, you may *importantize* your goal, but not *sacredize* it!

Rule No. 9: *Be interested in yourself and others.* One way to grow older gracefully is to take interest in the social world around you. As a human being, you are likely to feel happy in the company of others, at least some selected others. You may even like to help others in some way. If so, you can help others by yourself or by joining an organization of your choice. Suppose you are keen on giving free coaching in mathematics to schoolchildren who are weak in that subject and cannot afford to pay the fee of a private tutor. In that case, you may teach mathematics to poor schoolchildren free of charge. Or, you may join an organization dedicated to offering free coaching in all subjects to poor schoolchildren. In fact, you can do many things for others with a view to improving their miserable lot. This kind of social work will add to your happiness too.

However, you had better remain alert when you sincerely take interest in others and take pains to help them. Gradually, you may start believing that the more devotedly you help others, the more is your worth as a human being. This can be dangerous in two ways. First, some individuals or organizations may begin to exploit you and get you do a lot of more work than you are willing to do. Second, if you hanker after the praise and appreciation of such people, you may feel worthless unless you meet their demands.

Therefore, it is better to remember the two rules of morality given by Ellis. First, *be kind to yourself, love yourself and safeguard your own interest.* Second, *never harm others unnecessarily.* Emotionally healthy people wisely put their own interest at least little above the interest of others. They enjoy helping others, but not at the cost of their own well-being and happiness.

Rule No. 10: *Don't expect heaven on earth.* You may strive to grow gracefully by following many paths you prefer. Don't entertain any utopian idea of living a perfectly happy life free from all emotional disturbances, interpersonal tensions and other hassles. If you nurture any utopian expectations, you will soon get disillusioned with the idea of growing older gracefully. Strive for a reasonably happy and creative life, but keep in mind that probably nobody can live a blissfully happy life on earth.

Obviously, this rule is consistent with the rational and realistic philosophy of life that Ellis has been preaching throughout his life. It was his 93rd birthday on 27 September 2006. How far did he himself follow his own the rules of ageing gracefully? Remarkably well! Even today, we can unreservedly repeat what Daniel N. Wiener (1988) said about him: 'his own life is his message!'

REBT in Industry

REBT has been implemented successfully in the organizational context as well (Lange & Grieger, 1993). It has been widely used in employee development, organizational development, business consultation and other areas of people management. It is used to help people with their everyday problems and to enable them to be happier and more productive.

Employees in the organization are not only expected to do the assigned work but *must* also meet the workplace challenges successfully. REBT helps them in developing emotional muscle to face these challenges. There are many occasions when employees encounter emotional and other difficulties in the workplace. They needlessly upset themselves about the way of their colleagues, boss and subordinates, which they cannot change. They rant and rave about 'impossible' work conditions and thereby make them worse. They demand for perfectionistic work. They cannot stand predictably frustrating circumstances. REBT helps the employees in tackling day-to-day psychological problems and gaining effective self-management. It equips them in rational decision-making, constructive interpersonal relationships and effective self-management.

Ellis had done a large amount of work with business leaders, industry and government in his psychotherapeutic practice. He gave many talks and workshops to businessmen and wrote the first book on REBT for people working in organizations, *Executive Leadership: A Rational Approach* (Ellis, 1972a). This book is a training guide for executives and provides rational and effective solutions to their problems. It teaches them to be powerful at handling themselves and handling organizational affairs by fully accepting themselves and acquiring a clear perception of reality.

Ellis' valuable work in the industrial world has been taken ahead successfully by his associates. Some of the notable names are J.P. Anderson, R.C. Diedrich, D.J. Dimattia, R.R. Kilburg, P. Kirby, J. Sherin and L. Caigrer. They have implemented REBT in numerable fields such as leadership training, organizational crisis, executive coaching, effective performance, organizational management, etc. They have executed a number of training programmes based on the REBT model. In these programmes, trainees are helped to focus on problem solving and to get rid of rigidity of thoughts.

Models of Executive Coaching

Many of the executive coaching models include behaviour change as a fundamental aspect of their process (Kiel et al., 1996; Kilburg, 2000). A well-known model of executive coaching based on REBT is called 'rational emotive behavioural coaching' (REBC). It was developed by Kirby (1993). It has a five-step process that incorporates the REBT model into behaviour change stage at of the coaching process.

In the first step, the coach and client define the problem altogether. activating event (A) and consequences (C) are decided at this step. For example, the executive has a demanding workload and he is anxious for slipping deadlines due to it. Here, the demanding workload is 'A' and the inability to pay attention to the important task (behaviour) and the anxiety towards the work (emotion) is 'C'. Truly speaking, his problem is practical. He is not able to solve it as his main problem is surrounded by his anxiety. The coach empowers him to search for available alternatives to meet his deadlines with the existing workload. One of the sensible alternative is to delegate some work to subordinates. However, this executive doesn't apply this alternative as he gets anxious that his credibility is at stake if his subordinates commit mistakes. As this alternative is the best available amongst all, the coach helps him to concentrate more on it and review it.

The second step involves detection of irrational beliefs underlying the dysfunctional behaviour of the client. Here, the coach tries to find out the client's absolutistic demands, that is, *musts* and *shoulds*. This step is difficult and thereby takes more time than the first one. In example cited previously, the executive's irrational belief is 'if I want *perfect* work, I *must* do it by myself'.

The third step aims at behavioural change. The irrational belief detected in the second step is challenged at this step. The coach works with the client to change his absolutistic thinking into preferential thinking. This step is deeper than the other steps. The coach in this cited example will provoke the executive to dispute his own belief by asking a series of Socratic questions to himself. For example, what do I mean by perfect work? What is the perfect definition of perfectionism? Where has it written? How am I so sure that my definition is correct? Is my work perfect each and every time? With the help of these questions, the coach tries to eradicate irrational belief from his client. He also assists him developing rational belief as substitute. For example, the work can be done well by others as well as myself or others are fallible human beings and even if they commit mistakes, it is not awful and horrible.

The fourth step involves monitoring the client's progress in disputing irrational beliefs and replacing them with rational beliefs. The coach closely observes if the client has actually implemented the chosen alternative. In the cited example, the coach tries to verify if the executive has actually delegated his work. If he has not delegated, the earlier steps are again reviewed. At this step, the client is engaged in regular practice of REBC method and techniques.

At the fifth and final step, the coach evaluates the client's behavioural change. The client is helped for working on other irrational beliefs and the coach guides him in eliminating them.

This model is successfully applied on executives who have performance issues, anger management issues, fear of confrontation and LFT (Sherin & Caiger, 2004).

REBT: Limitations and Critique

REBT, like all other psychotherapies, has been subject to criticism. Ellis was criticized heavily on various claims that he made about REBT. Ellis also countered the major points through his writings from time to time (Ellis, 1976). He also edited the book, *Theoretical and Empirical*

Foundations of Rational-Emotive Therapy (Ellis & Whiteley, 1979), and tried to respond to major objections brought by his critics. However, some of the objections raised on REBT are still unanswered or not justified satisfactorily by Ellis or his associates. They are considered in this book as limitations of REBT. These are precisely summarised here.

1. **Lack of scientific evidence:** Unlike behaviouristic or client-centred therapies, REBT is not well grounded in empirical research. It is difficult to verify the evidence of some of its concepts. Most of the REBT statements offered are very ambiguously related to research data or are not supported at all. Hence, REBT is based upon many assumptions concerning the nature of man and about the aetiology of psychological disturbances. Unless and until not backed by strong research, they cannot be considered scientific.

Besides, many of the outcome studies presented by Ellis to support REBT are strictly speaking not REBT outcome studies. They fall under a variety of rubrics, such as, cognitive therapy, self-instructional training, cognitive behaviour therapy and cognitive restructuring (DiGiuseppe, Miller & Trexler, 1976). There is a scarcity of research done exclusively on REBT. In short, Ellis' claim that REBT is supported by large numbers of well-designed scientific studies is fallacious (Ewart & Thoresen, 1979).

In this connection, it is better not to forget what Dr Daniel N. Wiener (1988) says about Ellis' neglect of scientific research. His observation is that although Ellis believed in scientific research, he himself had not done much research. What could be the cause of this discrepancy between his belief and practice? Ellis had given some reasons for not having done much research. For instance, he said that he could not get time or financial support to do research. However, it seems that the real cause is that his main interests had always been different. He enjoyed the role of a teacher and propagandist and he was certainly at his best when he was faithful to his self-chosen role. Hence, there is a reason to agree with Dr Wiener's comment that Ellis was more of a persuader or propagandist than the researcher.

2. **Ambiguous theory:** Critics proclaim that REBT theory is imprecise and general (Meichenbaum, 1979). The concepts offered in REBT theory are too naïve and simplistic. For example, self-talk is the key concept used in REBT. It proposes that humans talk to themselves (self-talk) before they get emotionally disturbed (consequence).

There is no objective evidence to believe this proposal. To reply to this criticism, Ellis says that humans talk to continuously themselves, even before disturbance, during disturbance and after disturbance. This claim is also not supported by any strong scientific evidence. Some researchers argue that most of the internal dialogue to which Ellis referred seemed to have followed, and not preceded, emotional disturbance. The so-called internal dialogue seemed to be more like a set of rationalizations designed to explain the reactions.

3. **Untestable hypotheses:** REBT consists of a set of hypotheses that need to be tested under different conditions. Ellis tried to review and interpret objectively evidence relevant to 32 hypotheses of REBT (Ellis, 1979b). However, this review also became the subject of criticism (Mahoney, 1979) as one does not come away with the sense of a model or theory at all after testing these hypotheses. Instead, it presents a collection of loosely related and poorly elucidated propositions. Researchers (Ewart & Thoresen, 1979, pp. 193–202) find that most of these hypotheses Ellis put forward and the evidence he cited in their favour do not contribute a great deal to therapeutic theory or practice. This is because (a) some hypotheses are so vague they could not possibly be tested in their present form; (b) some, while testable, do not seem very informative; (c) important instances of negative findings are not explained; (d) the relationship of certain predictions to REBT theory is ambiguous; (e) there are apparent inconsistencies among predictions; (f) several hypotheses seem indistinguishable from ones put forward by many other theories; and (g) in those few instances where distinctive and specific predictions are made, little or no research evidence is offered on their behalf.

4. **Confirmatory bias:** Though Ellis had presented impressive numbers of studies to support the theory of REBT, he was criticized for presenting selective data. Critics (Meichenbaum, 1979, pp. 174–176) argue that Ellis had focused only on confirmatory studies and omitted non-confirmatory critical studies. This is because a number of studies Ellis cited had been appropriately criticized and their data had been severely challenged.

Critics (Mahoney, 1979, pp. 177–180) therefore objected to Ellis for displaying confirmatory bias in his review. That is, he selectively emphasized those studies which supported REBT and disregarded the remainder. This leads to the practice of affirming the consequent—an illogical inference in which a true conclusion is used to defend a true premise (Mahoney, 1976; Weimer, 1977).

5. **Over-inclusivity:** The core of REBT is its cognitive emphasis. From its inception, it emphasized the process of changing human emotions and behaviour by reason and intellect. Its original title, 'rational therapy', was appropriate in that sense. Ellis began with a system of rational therapy but gradually has added so much to it and became so general that it lost its own identity. He incorporated emotive and behavioural in its title to show that not only cognition but it also empathizes even emotion and behaviour. This inclusion accommodates the entire gamut of 'humanism' to 'behaviourism'. The list of techniques used and taught by the REBT therapist includes most of those which might be used by eclectic therapists who are not devoted to any particular theory (Wiener, 1988). Hence, REBT is now indistinguishable from most action-oriented eclectic disciplines. As a result, REBT is unable to hold its cognitive exclusivism which was its core.

In this context, Paul Meehl's comment in his foreword to Ellis' biography (Wiener, 1988) is noteworthy. He commented that it is perhaps more important to Ellis to push his main points at the risk of oversimplification than to try to put everything together. For instance, Freud plus Pavlov plus Ellis plus Skinner and goodness knows what all into one integrated package.

6. **Lack of research on forms of REBT:** Meichenbaum (1979, pp. 174–176) and Mahoney (1979, pp. 177–180) argue that though Ellis made a distinction between elegant and inelegant REBT, it is rarely used in actual therapy. Most of the REBT therapists use inelegant or general REBT. Ellis or his associates were not able to produce satisfactory answer to why REBT is frequently used inelegantly. Moreover, very little research is done on elegant REBT. So it becomes difficult to testify the difference.

7. **Overemphasis on life philosophy:** REBT aims at changing life or generalized faulty philosophy of person. According to some researchers, philosophy can be consequential and not necessarily be generalized. It can vary from person to person or also it can be generalized on some occasions and consequential on other occasions for one person. It can also be task specific. This fact is ignored in REBT. For example, a child procrastinates in studies.

REBT therapist concludes that he has LFT philosophy. That means his irrational belief falls in third category of beliefs, that is, world *must* be easy. It is possible that same child has passion for stamp collection and he pursues this hobby with great tolerance. That means it is wrong to conclude his life philosophy only on the basis of his behaviour in studies because he has LFT philosophy only on one particular occasion. Hence, it is task specific and not generalized. REBT needs to take into consideration task-specific or consequential philosophy along with generalized philosophy.

8. **Unrealistic unconditional acceptance:** Ellis (1979b) accepted that virtually no studies exist that investigate the validity of unconditional self and there would consists of no rating of oneself or essence, with the exception of one partially confirming study (Miller, 1976). He further suggested that more studies of this subject would seem called for.

While reviewing this view, Fredric Kleiner (1976) commented that the concept of unconditional acceptance consists of no rating of one's self or essence is itself is unrealistic. So it is difficult to conduct studies on unrealistic concept. Following unconditional acceptance in practical life is virtually impossible. To certain extent, one's self or essence could be implemented by enlightened masters such as Zen Masters, yoga masters, Tibetan Tulkus or Lamas. It is difficult to find a single common man who follows this concept in his life. Kleiner (1976, p. 189) further commented, 'In my experience I have never met anyone who is totally devoid of rating him or herself, and that includes Ellis himself!'

9. **Mysticism of self-worth:** REBT makes distinction between performance and worth. The reasoning behind is that we can measure or evaluate our performance or behaviour, but our intrinsic value or worth cannot be really measured because our being includes their becoming. Ellis found out elegant solution by believing that an individual does not have to rate himself, esteem himself or have any self-measurement or self-concept whatsoever (Ellis, 1973).

Critics object that this reasoning is lame on scientific criterion. The universally accepted criterion of existence given by Thurstone is that 'whatever exists, it *should* be measured in principle'. If there is no measurement, we cannot differentiate between existence and non-existence. By applying the same criterion to self-worth, there are two alternatives. If it exists, it *should* be measured or it doesn't exist, there is no question of measurement. Ellis doesn't accept any of this alternative and say that self-worth exists but cannot be measured (beyond measurement). This is unscientific and leads to mysticism. If there is no measurement, logically it doesn't exist. To support such mystical concepts weakens REBT's scientific foundation.

10. **Criticism on self-worth:** If self-worth comes under the purview of measurement, to rate one's self as 'good' or 'bad' will depend on the success or failure of one's performance, which will lead to permanent insecurity. The idea of personal worth used in REBT is intrinsic which is without rating. Some researchers challenged this idea of intrinsic personal in the context of characteristics of mentally healthy person described by Ellis (Ellis, Abrams & Abrams, 2009). One of the characteristic is acceptance of uncertainty. It suggests that an emotionally healthy person acknowledges and accepts the fact that we live in a world of probability and chance, where absolute certainties don't, and probably never will, exist. Researchers argue that if the person is ready to accept uncertainty of the world around us, it would not be difficult for him to accept uncertainty even of his own worth. He needs to accept that like changes in the world, even the personal worth will also go up and down according to the performance. Therefore, there is no need to keep the idea of personal worth to be intrinsic. It can be used extrinsically and the rating can be given to it.

Another criticism is on it that it is a doctrine of incompetent and inefficient people. If the person is considered worthwhile just because he exists, everybody gets the same value irrespective of their performances. In that case, there will be no distinction between competent and incompetent people. It will lead to the promotion of incompetence. Ellis or his associates could not give justifiable answer to this criticism.

11. **Procrustean approach:** REBT is criticized as having procrustean approach to treatment. 'Procrustean bed' is a scheme or pattern into which someone or something is arbitrarily forced. Lazarus (1989), creator of multimodal therapy noted that he has seen many clients in REBT who did not appear to subscribe any of the musturbatory categories Ellis has identified in his writings. But Ellis and REBT therapist tend 'to employ procrustean manoeuvers' fitting the client to 11 or 12 preconceived beliefs. Ellis had not offered any response to this charge.

12. **Subjective terms:** Many behaviourists criticize REBT and cognitive therapy for the usage of a number of subjective terms, for example, frequently used terms in REBT such as awfulization or LFT. These terms are very subjective and their meaning differs from person to person. In REBT, awful is assumed to be more than 100 per cent bad, but the person might not feel more than 100 per cent bad. It impairs the objectivity of the theory.

Last Words

Ellis had epistemophilic personality. He strived to seek answer for every objection raised against REBT. This can be identified from his profuse writing on reviews on REBT. He was relentlessly ruminating over the criticism to which he could not reply satisfactorily. Until his last breadth at 93, he was modifying personality theory of REBT, the result of which was creation of his book, *Personality Theories: Critical Perspectives* (Ellis, Abrams & Abrams, 2009), published after his death. It reveals his rework on ABC framework. His persistence and undogmatic approach are clearly indicated in this work.

When Ellis was in hospital, his wife Debbie asked him a question, 'what would you like your supporters to do for your speedy recovery?' He replied,

'Those wish me to recover soon, I would like them to live rationally. I would be happy if they do not lose their freedom even in the case of toughest situation. If more and more people embrace rational philosophy of life, I would definitely recover soon'.

Kudos to Ellis for his great work, passion and the revolution he brought in psychology by giving birth to REBT!

References

Alcoholic Anonymous. (2013). *Alcoholic Anonymous: The Story of How Many Thousands of Men and Women Have Recovered from Alcoholism* (*The Big Book*, 4th ed.). New York, NY: AA World Services, Inc.

DiGiuseppe, R.A., Miller, N.J., & Trexler, L.D. (1976). A review of rational-emotive psychotherapy outcome studies. In A. Ellis & J.M. Whiteley (Eds), *Theoretical and*

Empirical Foundations of Rational-Emotive Therapy (pp. 218–235). Monterey, CA: Brooks/Cole.

Ellis, A. (1951). *The Folklore of Sex* (Rev. ed., 1961). New York, NY: Grove Press.

———. (1954). *The American Sexual Tragedy*. New York, NY: Twayne. [Rev. ed. (1962). New York: Lyle Stuart and Grove Press.]

———. (1956a). New light on masturbation. *The Independent* 51, 4.

———. (1956b). *The Psychology of Sex Offenders*. Springfield, IL: Thomas.

———. (1960). *The Art and Science of Love*. New York, NY: Lyle Stuart.

———. (1963a). Is the vaginal orgasm a myth? *The International Journal of Sexology/ Liaison, 1*(9), 2–4.

———. (1963b). *Sex and the Single Man*. New York: Lyle Stuart.

———. (1963). *The Intelligent Woman's Guide to Man Hunting*. New York: Lyle Stuart and Dell Publishing. [Rev. ed. (1979). *The Intelligent Woman's Guide to Dating and Mating*. Secaucus, NJ: Lyle Stuart.]

———. (1964). A guide to rational homosexuality. *Drum: Sex in Perspective, 4*(8), 8–12.

———. (1965a). *The Case for Sexual Liberty*. Tucson, AZ: Seymour Press.

———. (1965b). *Homosexuality: Its Causes and Cure*. New York, NY: Lyle Stuart.

———. (1969, November). Teaching emotional education in the classroom. *School Health Review,* 10–13.

———. (1972a). *Executive Leadership: A Rational-Emotive Approach*. New York, NY: Institute for Rational-Emotive Therapy.

———. (1972b). *The Civilized Couple's Guide to Extramarital Adventures*. New York, NY: Pinnacle Books.

———. (1972c). *The Sensuous Person: Critique and Corrections*. Secaucus, NY: Lyle Stuart.

———. (1973). *Humanistic Psychotherapy: The Rational Emotive Approach* (p. 65). New York, NY: Julian Press.

———. (1976). Answering a critique of rational-emotive therapy. *Canadian Journal of Counselling and Psychotherapy, 10*(2), 56–59.

———. (1976). *Sex and the Liberated Man*. Secaucus, NJ: Lyle Stuart.

———. (1977). How I became interested in sexology and sex therapy. In B. Bullough, V.L. Bullough, M.A. Fithian, W.E. Hartman, & R.S. Klein (Eds.), *Personal Stories of How I Got Into Sex* (pp. 131–40). Amherst, NY: Prometheus Book.

———. (1979a). Foreword. In M. De Martino, *Human Autoerotic Practices* (pp. 9–18). New York, NY: Human Sciences Press.

———. (1979b). Rational-emotive therapy: Research and conceptual support. In A. Ellis & J.M. Whiteley (Eds.), *Theoretical and Empirical Foundations of Rational-Emotive Therapy* (pp. 101–173). Monterey, CA: Brooks/Cole.

———. (1992). *How to Age With Style*. Cassette Recording. New York, NY: Institute for Rational-Emotive Therapy.

———. (2003). *Sex Without Guilt in the 21st Century* (pp. 121–128). New Jersey: Barricade Books.

Ellis, A., & Abarbanel, A. (1961). (Eds). *Encyclopedia of Sexual Behaviour*. New York, NY: Howthorne.

Ellis, A., & Mclerney, J., DiGiuseppe, R., & Yeager, R. (1988). *Rational-Emotive Therapy with Alcoholics and Substance Abusers*. Elmsford, NY: Pergamon.

Ellis, A., & Velten, E. (1992). *When AA doesn't Work for You: Rational Steps to Quitting Alcohol*. Fort Lee, NJ: Barricade.

Ellis, A., & Velten, E. (1998). *Optimal Aging: Get Over Getting Older*. Chicago: Open Court.

Ellis, A., & Whiteley, J.M. (1979). *Theoretical and Empirical Foundations of Rational-Emotive Therapy.* Monterey, CA: Brooks/Cole.

Ellis, A., Wolfe, J.L., & Moseley, S. (1966). *How to Prevent Your Child from Becoming a Neurotic Adult.* New York: Crown, 1966. [Paperback ed., (1972). *How to Raise an Emotionally Healthy, Happy Child.* North Hollywood: Wilshire Books.]

Ellis, A. & Wilde, J. (2001). *Case Studies in REBT with Children and Adolescents.* New York: Prentice-Hall.

Ellis, A. Abrams, M., & Abrams, L. (2009). *Personality Theories: Critical Perspectives.* Thousand Oaks, CA: SAGE.

Ewart, C.K., & Thoresen, C.T. (1979). The rational-emotive manifesto. In A. Ellis, & J.M. Whiteley (Eds.), *Theoretical and Empirical Foundations of Rational-Emotive Therapy* (pp. 193–202). Monterey, CA: Brooks/Cole.

Gerald, M., & Eyman, W. (1980). *Thinking Straight and Talking Sense: An Emotional Education Programme.* New York: Institute for Rational-Emotive Therapy.

Kiel, F., Rimmer, E., Williams, K., & Doyle, M. (1996). Coaching at the top. *Consulting Psychology Journal: Practice and Research, 48,* 67–77.

Kilburg, R.R. (2000). *Executive Coaching: Developing Managerial Wisdom on a World of Chaos.* Washington, DC: American Psychological Association.

Kinsey, A.C., Pomeroy, W.B., & Martin, C. (1948). *Sexual Behavior in the Human Male.* Philadelphia: Saunders.

Kinsey, A.C., Pomeroy, W.B., & Martin, C.,& Bell, A. (1953). *Sexual Behavior in the Human Female.* Philadelphia: Saunders.

Kirby, P. (1993). RET counseling: Application in management and executive development. *Journal of Rational-Emotive & Behavior Therapy, 11*(1), 7–18.

Kleiner, F.B. (1976). Commentary on Albert Ellis' article. In A. Ellis & J.M. Whiteley (Eds.), *Theoretical and Empirical Foundations of Rational-Emotive Therapy* (pp. 188–92). Monterey, CA: Brooks/Cole.

Lange, A., & Grieger, R. (1993). Integrating RET into management consulting and training. *Journal of Rational-Emotive & Cognitive-Behavior Therapy, 11*(1), 51–57.

Lazarus, A.A. (1989). *The Practice of Multimodal Therapy.* Baltimore: Johns Hopkins University Press.

Mahoney, M.J. (1976). *Scientist as Subject: The Psychological Imperative.* Cambridge, Mass: Ballinger.

———. (1979). A critical analysis of rational-emotive theory and therapy. In A. Ellis & J.M. Whiteley (Eds.), *Theoretical and Empirical Foundations of Rational-Emotive Therapy* (pp. 177–80). Monterey, CA: Brooks/Cole.

Meichenbaum, D. (1979). Dr Ellis, please stand up! In A. Ellis, & J.M. Whiteley (Eds.), *Theoretical and Empirical Foundations of Rational-Emotive Therapy* (pp. 174–76). Monterey, CA: Brooks/Cole.

Miller, T.W. (1976). An exploratory investigation comparing self-esteem with self-acceptance in reducing social evaluating anxiety (Doctoral dissertation). Syracuse University, Syracuse, New York.

Phadke. K.M. (1999). *Adhunik Sanjivani* (pp. 290–317). Mumbai: Tridal Prakashan.

Pillay, A.P., & Ellis, A. (1953). *Sex, society and the individual* (p. 488). Bombay: *International Journal of Sexology, 488.*

Salter, A. (1949). *Conditioned Reflex Therapy.* New York: Creative Age Press.

Sherin, J., & Caiger, L. (2004). Rational-emotive behaviour therapy: A behavioural change model for executive coaching? *Consulting Psychology Journal: Practice and Research, 56*(4), 225–33.

Trimpey, J. (1992). *The Small Book: A Revolutionary Alternative for Overcoming Alcohol and Drug Dependence*. New York: Delacorate Press.

Trimpey, J. (1996). *Rational Recovery: The New Care for Substance Addiction*. New York: Pocket Books.

Weimer, W.B. (1977). *Psychology and the Conceptual Foundations of Science*. Hillsdale, NJ: Erlbaum.

Wiener, D.N. (1988). *Albert Ellis: Passionate Skeptic*. New York: Praeger.

Weinberg, J.R. (1975). *AA: An Interpretation for the Nonbeliever*. Minnesota: Hazelden Foundation.

Further Readings

Dames, J. (1991). Counseling in the classroom: Interview with Albert Ellis. *Journal of Rational-Emotive and Cognitive-Behavior Therapy, 9*(4), 247–263.

DiMattia, D., & Lega, L. (1990). (Eds.). *Will the Real Albert Ellis Please Stand Up?* Anecdotes by his colleagues, students, and friends celebrating his 75th birthday. New York, NY: Albert Ellis Institute.

Dryden, W. (Ed.). (1990). *The Essential Albert Ellis*. New York, NY: Springer.

Ellis, A. (1965). *Suppressed: Seven Key Essays Publishers Dared Not Print*. Chicago: New Classics House.

———. (1976). Nobody need feel ashamed or guilty about anything. In S. Kopp (Ed.), *The Naked Therapist*. San Diego: Edits Publishers.

———. (1979). Rejoinder: Elegant and inelegant RET. In A. Ellis & J.M. Whitley (Eds.), *Theoretical and Empirical Foundations of RET* (pp. 240–267). New York, NY: Brunner.

———. (1992). Are gays and lesbians emotionally disturbed? *The Humanist, 52*(5), 33–35.

———. (1997). Using rational emotive behavior therapy techniques to cope with disability. *Professional Psychology: Research and Practice, 28*(1), 17–22.

———. (2003a). *Ask Albert Ellis*. Atascadero, CA: Impact Publishers.

———. (2003b). *Sex Without Guilt in the Twenty-First Century*. Fort Lee, NJ: Barricade Books.

———. (2004a). *REBT: It Works for Me – It Works for You*. New York, NY: Prometheus Books.

———. (2004b). *The Road to Tolerance: The Philosophy of REBT*. New York, NY: Prometheus Books.

Greco, K. (November 2000). Aging with rational emotive therapy: A window of opportunity? *Pique*, 1–2.

Joshi, A. (2009). *Mee Albert Ellis*. Mumbai: Shabd Publication.

Lembo J.M. (1974). *Help Yourself*. Niles, IL: Argus Communications.

Phadke, K.M., & Chulani, V. (1998). *Liberation from Addictions*. Mumbai: Himalaya Publishing House.

Weinrach, S. (1980). Unconventional therapist: Albert Ellis. *The Personnel and Guidance Journal, 59*(3), 152–160.

Wessler, R.L. (1987). Listening to oneself: Cognitive appraisal therapy. In W. Dryden (Ed.), *Key Cases in Psychotherapy* (pp. 176–212). London, UK: Croom-Helm.

Appendices

Appendix I

The REBT Disputation Form (Practice)

- Fill in Section 'C'
- Write down 2 criteria of rational thinking
- Fill in section 'A'
- Fill in section 'B'
- Fill in section 'DA'
- Fill in section 'DB'
- Fill in section 'RB'
- Fill in section 'E'

Section A: Facts and Events	Section DA: Is It Factual?	
Section B : Irrational Self-talk	Disputation of Beliefs (DB)	Rational Beliefs (RB)
IB1	DB1	RB1
IB2	DB2	RB2

IB3	DB3	RB3
IB4	DB4	RB4
IB5	DB5	RB5
IB6	DB6	RB6

Section C: Emotions	Important Criteria for Rational Thinking 1. *Factual:* Is this thought based on fact or reality? 2. *Functional:* Is this thought likely to help me to undertake any constructive action?
Section E: Effective Philosophy	

Appendix II

The REBT Disputation Form (Solved)

- Fill in Section 'C'
- Write down 2 criteria of rational thinking
- Fill in section 'A'
- Fill in section 'B'
- Fill in section 'DA'
- Fill in section 'DB'
- Fill in section 'RB'
- Fill in section 'E'

Section A: Facts & Events	Section DA: Is it Factual?	
My subordinate has refused to do the work which I asked him to do so.	Yes. What I have written in Section A records the actual event objectively.	
Section B: Irrational Self-talk	**Disputation of Beliefs (DB)**	**Rational Beliefs (RB)**
IB1	**DB1**	**RB1**
1. How could he do so? (Rhetorical question— underlying assumption is that he *should* not do so.)	1. Is there any compulsion/ rule why he *should* not do so? (*Factual*) 2. Are there any absolute necessitates in human behaviour? (*Factual*) 3. Is he not free to behave as he wishes to? (*Factual*) 4. Is there any law of the universe which compels him to behave in any specific way? (*Factual*) 5. Where is it written that subordinate *should* not refuse the work? (*Factual*) 6. Who controls his brain, he or you? (*Factual*) 7. Is there any way to control other person's behaviour? (*Factual*)	1. It would be better/good if he has not done so, but there is no evidence to say that he *should* have not done so. 2. He is free to behave as he wishes to, even if he is my subordinate. 3. No law of the universe compels him to behave in any specific way. 4. Though I wish/expect strongly that he would not have refused my work, there is no reason to say that why he has not refused. 5. I can influence/teach/preach/ guide/advise other person but cannot control other person's behaviour totally. 6. Suppose there is a technique by which I can control other people's behaviour, I will not like if some other person using the same technique on me as

(Continued)

(Continued)

	8. Suppose there is a technique by which I can control other people's behaviour, how would I like some other person using the same technique on me? (*Factual*) 9. As a matter of fact, he did refuse my work. Is it not absurd to say that he *should* not have done so, what he actually did? (*Factual*) 10. Am I not denying the reality when he actually did so? (*Factual*) 11. Is this thinking going to help me to change his behaviour? (*Functional*)	I am free individual. I will not like of getting deprived of my freedom. Similarly, I will not deprive other person from his freedom. 7. It is absurd to say that he *should* not have done so, what he actually did. So by saying so, I am denying the reality. 8. This thinking is not going to help me to change his behaviour. So, I will focus my attention on the thought that how I will persuade him next time for changing his behaviour.
IB2 2. He always behaves in this manner.	**DB2** 1. Always? In each and every situation? How do you know? (*Factual*) 2. What is correct—he always behaves in this manner or most of the times? (*Factual*) 3. To say that he always behaves in this manner is not an exaggeration? (*Factual*) 4. How am I so sure/how am I so convinced that he will behave in similar manner in future too? (*Factual*) 5. Is this thought going to help me to take any constructive action for influencing him in future or am I condemning him forever? (*Functional*)	**RB2** 1. There is no evidence to say that he always behaves in this manner. 2. Most of the times, he behaves in this manner is a realistic statement. 3. I have no ability to predict future 100% right. Therefore, I cannot say that he will surely behave in similar manner in future too. 4. As I am not 100% sure about his future behaviour, I will accept that there might be a possibility that he may not repeat this behaviour in future. 5. If I accept that possibility, I will be able to concentrate on how to influence him next time; so that as far as possible, he will behave less frequently in that manner. 6. Condemning him will serve no purpose.

IB3	DB3	RB3
3. His refusal to do the work has lowered my status in the eyes of others & also in my own eyes.	1. How am I so sure that the refusal from one subordinate has lowered my status? (*Factual*) 2. What do I mean by lowering down the status? (*Factual*) 3. Is there any universal behaviour which if somebody follows will surely increase or lower down the status? (*Factual*) 4. Does lowering down the status depend only on subordinate's refusal? (*Factual*) 5. If he obeys me, can I say surely that my status has increased? (*Factual*) 6. Suppose my status lowers down in their eyes, what calamity is going to fall on me? (*Factual*) 7. Suppose my status has lowered in the eyes of others, does it mean that I also have to lower down my status in my own eyes? Is my status so fragile like a glass of water? (*Factual*) 8. What compels me to do so? (*Factual*) 9. Which law of the universe compels me to seek approval from others for maintenance of my status? (*Factual*) 10. What is my goal? Increasing my status in my own eyes/in the eyes of others or getting the work done? (*Functional*)	1. There is no evidence to say that the status of all the people lowers down if their subordinates refuse to do their work. 2. There is no universal behaviour which if somebody follows will surely increase or lower down the status. 3. If one of my subordinates obeys me once, my status does not increase. Similarly, if he refuses to do my work, it does not decrease. 4. Therefore, I conclude that somebody's acceptance or refusal of my work is no way related to my status. 5. Suppose my status lowers down in other's eyes, no calamity is going to fall on me. It will be disadvantageous; but it will certainly not be a catastrophic situation. 6. My status is not so fragile like a glass of water that eyes of the others will damage it. 7. I do not depend so much on other's approval for maintenance of my status. 8. If others lower down my status in their eyes, there is no compulsion on me that I have to show agreement with them. I still have a choice whether to lower it down or not in my own eyes. 9. My goal is not to maintain my status but to get my work done.

(Continued)

IB4	DB4	RB4
4. How will I get my work done if all other subordinates start disobeying me?	1. Do I mean to say that if one of my subordinates disobeys me once, *all* will start disobeying me? How do I know? *(Factual)* 2. Why will all start doing that way? Where is the evidence? *(Factual)* 3. Is it not an exaggeration? *(Factual)* 4. How am I so sure about the future that all of them behave in a similar manner? *(Factual)* 5. Is their behaviour totally in my hands? *(Factual)* 6. What is in my control, their behaviour or my behaviour? 7. Why am I concentrating on the facts that are beyond my control? 8. If few disobey me, isn't there a possibility that few others will obey me? *(Factual)* 9. Will all of them obey me if he obeys me? *(Factual)* 10. Suppose all of them start disobeying me, will it be really awful or disadvantageous? *(Factual)* 11. Suppose all of them start disobeying me, does my work gets stalled completely or some of the work I could still able to do? *(Factual)*	1. There is no reason to believe that if one of my subordinates disobeys me once, *all* will start disobeying me. 2. I have no evidence to prove that all will behave in a similar manner in future just because of the refusal of one of the subordinates. 3. Other's behaviour is not totally in my hands. 4. Instead of wasting my energy on controlling other's behaviour, which is beyond my control, I will concentrate on how will I change my behaviour which is in my control. 5. If few disobey me, there is a possibility that few others still obey me. 6. Whether others will obey me or not does not totally depend on one of my subordinates' behaviour. 7. There is no guarantee that they will obey me if he obeys me. Similarly, there is no guarantee that they will disobey me if he disobeys me. 8. Suppose all of them start disobeying me, still it will not be really awful. It will be disadvantageous. 9. Suppose all of them start disobeying me, it is an exaggeration to say that my work will get completely stalled. Some of the work I could still able to do. 10. Under that condition too, I still have a choice to bear the circumstances without whining.

	12. Suppose all of them start disobeying me and some of my work gets stalled, what else can I do in these circumstances rather than to bear this? (*Factual*) 13. Under that condition too, am I fully choiceless? Do I still not have choice in those circumstances to bear it whiningly or without whiningly? (*Factual*) 14. Suppose all of them start disobeying me, what lesson will I learn about my methods of supervision? (*Functional*) 15. Is it not wise to think of techniques that I better adopt to prevent their disobedience rather than expressing helplessness? (*Functional*)	11. It is possible that I will review my methods of supervision& try to improve them. 12. I will try to adopt techniques which will prevent the disobedience of my subordinates rather than expressing helplessness.
IB5	**DB5**	**RB5**
5. He is an arrogant man; therefore, he *should* be condemned by all people in our company.	1. Is he arrogant man or is he behaving arrogantly now? (*Factual*) 2. By calling him an arrogant man, do I mean to say that he has always acted arrogantly, is acting arrogantly and will continue to act arrogantly until his death? (*Factual*) 3. Have I ever come across any such person? (*Factual*)	1. To say that he is an arrogant man is an exaggeration because by calling anybody an arrogant person indicates that he has always acted arrogantly, is acting arrogantly and will continue to act arrogantly until his death. 2. I have never come across any such person nor do I think any such human being could ever exist on this planet. 3. Perhaps he is like many other human beings who sometimes behave arrogantly and sometimes even politely.

(*Continued*)

(*Continued*)

	4. Do I think any such human being could have ever existed on this planet? 5. Just because somebody refuses to do the work given by me, does he become totally arrogant person? Is it not an overgeneralization? (*Factual*) 6. Even if he has refused to do the work, how am I going to calculate exact punishment to be imposed on him? (*Factual*) 7. Am I a judge of Supreme Court or God to decide exact punishment? (*Factual*) 8. If I label him an arrogant, am I not aggravating my problem in the future too? (*Functional*) 9. If I call him an arrogant man, will it not prevent me from establishing cordial relations with him in future? (*Functional*) 10. Will my problem of getting the work done really get over by condemning him? (*Functional*)	4. Just because somebody refuses to do the work given by me, I can say that he is behaving arrogantly. But he does not become *totally* arrogant person because of his one deed. Calling him totally arrogant is an overgeneralization. 5. I am not a judge of Supreme Court to decide or calculate exact punishment to be imposed on him for his refusal. 6. Judging him and saying that he is good or bad is not my job; perhaps it is a job of God. 7. By labelling him an arrogant person, I am closing down the opportunity to deal with him in future. 8. If I open this opportunity, I will try to develop cordial relations with him but, if I label him as an arrogant man, I will behave with him in an inimical manner. 9. If I behave in inimical manner, he may start behaving in a similar manner. Finally, it may end in taking revenge. 10. My problem of getting the work done is not going to get over by condemning him. Therefore, realistic conclusion is that I may like or dislike his behaviour, but I will neither praise nor dislike *him* as a totality.
IB6 6. I don't think I will ever learn to deal with such people.	**DB6** 1. *Ever?* How am I so sure? (*Factual*)	**RB6** 1. If I am not able to deal with one of my subordinates today, I am denying the possibility of bringing about a change in myself.

	2. Do I mean to say that if I am not able to deal with one of my subordinates today, I will *never* able to deal with him or people like him in future? (*Factual*) 3. Where is the evidence to predict that I will never be able to deal with such people? (*Factual*) 4. Then what do I mean by learning? Isn't learning mean to do something which I am not doing now? (*Functional*) 5. Will this thought help me in generating any method of tackling them in future? (*Functional*)	2. There is no evidence to predict that I will *never* be able to deal with such people in future. 3. As I am not 100% sure about my future behaviour, I will accept that there might be a possibility that I can deal with such people in future. 4. If I accept that possibility, I will be able to concentrate on how will I able to deal with such people next time. 5. Even if I am not able to deal with such people so far, I learn a lesson that some of the techniques I have used so far are not useful. I still have a further scope in future. 6. I will focus my attention on generating any method of tackling them in future.
Section C: **Emotions** Anger, Humiliation, Anxiety	Important Criteria for Rational Thinking 1. *Factual:* Is this thought based on fact or reality? 2. *Functional:* Will this thought help me to take any constructive action?	

Emotive Slogan: Sticks and stones may break my bones, but words will never hurt me.

Section E: Effective Philosophy
- I will differentiate behaviour form totality.
- I will not label totality.
- I will treat every individual as a unique example of human being.

Index

About the Authors

Anjali Joshi is a practising counselling psychologist and associate professor at Prin. W.N. Welingkar Institute of Management Development & Research, Mumbai, and has spent 22 years working in the field of education. Dr Joshi holds Master's degree in counselling psychology, MPhil in geriatric counselling, and PhD in REBT psychotherapy. She has delivered several lectures and conducted numerous workshops in organizations of repute, and conducts personal and group counselling programs, employee training programmes, corporate training programmes and weekend workshops on effective self-management through REBT. Dr Joshi was awarded the 'Young Doctoral Fellowship' by the Indian Council of Social Science Research (ICSSR), Ministry of Human Resource Development, New Delhi, for her doctoral work. She has published 90 articles and research papers in national and international journals. She writes both fiction and non-fiction, and has authored several books. Dr Joshi is a Linnaeus Palme (Sweden) scholar and a recipient of several awards such as 'Best Academic Performance', 'Best Mentor', 'Outstanding Achievement' and 'Best Literature' by Maharashtra Foundation and Maharashtra Sahitya Parishad.

K.M. Phadke is an Indian psychologist, practitioner and trainer in Rational Emotive Behaviour Therapy, with 45 years of rich experience in the fields of psychological education, research, training and consultation. He enjoys the unique distinction of being the first and only Indian psychologist to have earned the status of fellow and supervisor of the Albert Ellis Institute (AEI), New York, USA. Mr Phadke had extensive professional correspondence with Albert Ellis, which lasted for 36 years. This correspondence is considered one of the finest resources for REBT learners and is preserved in four volumes in the Archives of Columbia University. Mr Phadke has made original contributions to the theory and practice of REBT and was praised by Dr Ellis for his dedication and mastery over the subject. He has conducted scores of lectures and workshops at various business, industrial, educational, research, training and social organizations throughout India and has authored several books on REBT.